CHANTAY WATSON

Fit For Less

An Introduction To Simple At Home Exercises Requiring Less Equipment and Less Time, In Hopes of Motivating Middle-Aged Working Women to Stay Activate and Feel Good.

This book was professionally typeset on Reedsy.
Find out more at reedsy.com

Contents

INTRODUCTION

Welcome to Fit For Less, a brief guide to fitness for busy women reaching their middle age years. My name is C.L. Watson and I am excited to share with you some of my favorite exercises to do at home. I hope this book is seen as a starting point as a way for you to become more active and motivated by using simple moves that can be done with little equipment,and minimal time in the comfort of your own home.

A brief background about myself... I am a 45 year old full time working mother of two and have been married for 20 years to the love of my life. I have a degree in Physical Education and health and have spent the past 22 years coaching and teaching in my hometown. I stay active, as my job requires it, yet the older I get I find myself lacking motivation. When I am done working for the day the last thing I want to do is head to the gym and spend more hours of time away from my family. However, I find myself continually searching for simple ways to get fit.

As women age we experience so many changes in our bodies and I for one find it increasingly difficult to maintain my desired weight. There is this constant pressure of living up to the perfect image that we are all made to believe in through the media. I try to eat well and stay active yet always feel like I am working so hard to move forward only to find that I have taken two steps back. The lack of seeing results can be disheartening. The struggle is real!

Therefore, I have decided to give up on reaching some set standard and love the body image that I am. I fully believe that movement is integral to our overall health and well being, but it shouldn't have to take us away from our families or take up so much time. Maintaining a healthy lifestyle should be simple and make us feel good, not feel like more work.

Through a lot of searching I have found some exercises that I can easily do at home with little or no equipment. I can do these in a short amount of time in a variety of combinations to suit my desires for that day. Best of all, I can do them at home! I am hopeful that some of these ideas help you feel more motivated and know that exercise doesn't have to be hard.

Good luck on your journey!

DISCLAIMER

The exercises provided in this book are for educational and idea purposes only, in hopes of giving you a starting point to get motivated and more active. The information provided should not to be interpreted as a recommendation for a specific treatment plan, or course of action. Exercise does have its own inherent risks, and the exercises in this book,or any exercise program may result in injury. Possible risks can include but are not limited to: risk of injury, or aggravating a pre-existing condition. Exercise could result in over-exertion, muscle injury, rising or abnormal blood pressure. In more rare instances, exercise can lead to fainting, irregular heartbeat, and very rare instances of heart attack.

You should always consult with a physician or trained medical professional before beginning this or any exercise program. They will be able to provide you with appropriate exercise programs and safety precautions. The content of this book and advice presented are in no way intended as a substitute for medical consultation.

I disclaim any liability from and in connection with this program and how individuals choose to proceed and perform the suggested exercises. As is the case with any physical activity and any exercise routine, if at any point during your workout you begin to feel adverse effects such as dizziness or fainting. Or if you should experience any physical discomfort, stop what you are doing immediately and seek medical council from a physician.

TYPES OF EXERCISES

There are many types of exercises and it is important to remember that they are not all equal. Because of this, it is important to include a mix of exercise types into your routine. The following are four types of exercise that you may want to cycle through your workouts:

- **Strength training**

Weight training exercises that I like to do include the use of light weight dumbbells or kettle bells. I also like to do exercises that can be done with or without the addition of resistance bands to strengthen my core and extremities. Strength and resistance training is important for women as we age as they can help to not only reverse the loss of muscle mass, but can also help to slow down bone loss.

- **Aerobic/cardiovascular**

These exercises work on your endurance and should be maintained for at least 10 minutes. While doing this style of exercise you should notice an increase in your heart rate. While I do not necessarily choose to do most of these particular exercises at home, I still try to include them in my weekly routine. My favorite cardio exercise is walking! I speed up my pace for added benefit and to get that heart rate up. I like to walk where I can fit it in. This could be as simple as parking as far back in a lot as possible to force myself to get in the steps. I also like to get in a few laps on an outdoor track at work either during lunch or by arriving 10 minutes prior to the start of my workday. Swimming, Dancing and using an elliptical are also great aerobic options.

- **Stretching**

Stretching is so important. For one it just feels good. But more importantly, it is integral in helping us to increase and maintain our flexibility while also minimizing our risk of injury. When stretching please remember to listen to your body. The stretch should feel oh so good, not oh so ouch. If there is pain, your body is telling you that you are stretching too far and you should release or back off of the hold until a comfortable stretch is reached.

- **Balance**

As we age, there is an increased risk in falling. We do exercises that strengthen our core while also improving our balance in hopes that these risks are reduced. Standing on one foot is a very simple example of an exercise that can be used to help improve balance.

Remember that when we perform these exercises, they are not exclusive to one of the aforementioned categories. They often cross over. For instance, you can be doing an exercise that is focused on building strength, yet in the process is improving your balance or providing a muscle stretch. Likewise, aerobic exercise can build your strength along with endurance

STRETCHES

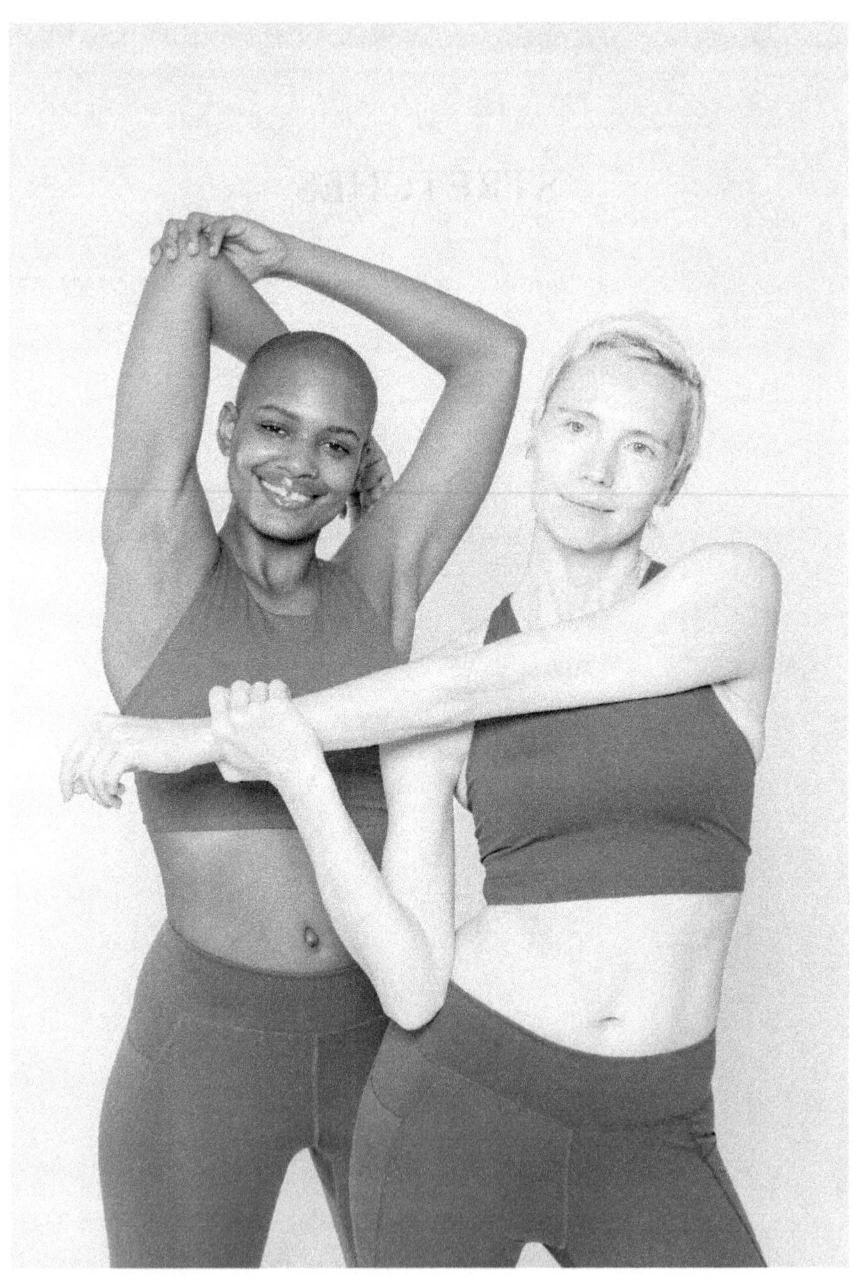

SEATED NECK RELEASE

I like to start with this stretch to relieve tension in my neck, but also feel the benefits in my shoulders and spine. Tension is often formed through the neck and shoulders from stress and by performing everyday repetitive activities.

To perform this stretch you can choose to do it in a standing or seated position.

- Standing: do so with feet shoulder width apart.
- Sitting: do so by lifting your chest and keeping your back in a straight line.
- Next: Choose a side to start with. For instance, if starting with the right side, slowly lower your right ear down to your right shoulder and maintain this position.
- If you would like to deepen this stretch use the hand on that same side to reach up and gently press your head toward the shoulder.
- After holding this stretch for 15-30 seconds, switch sides. Repeat the steps if you choose.

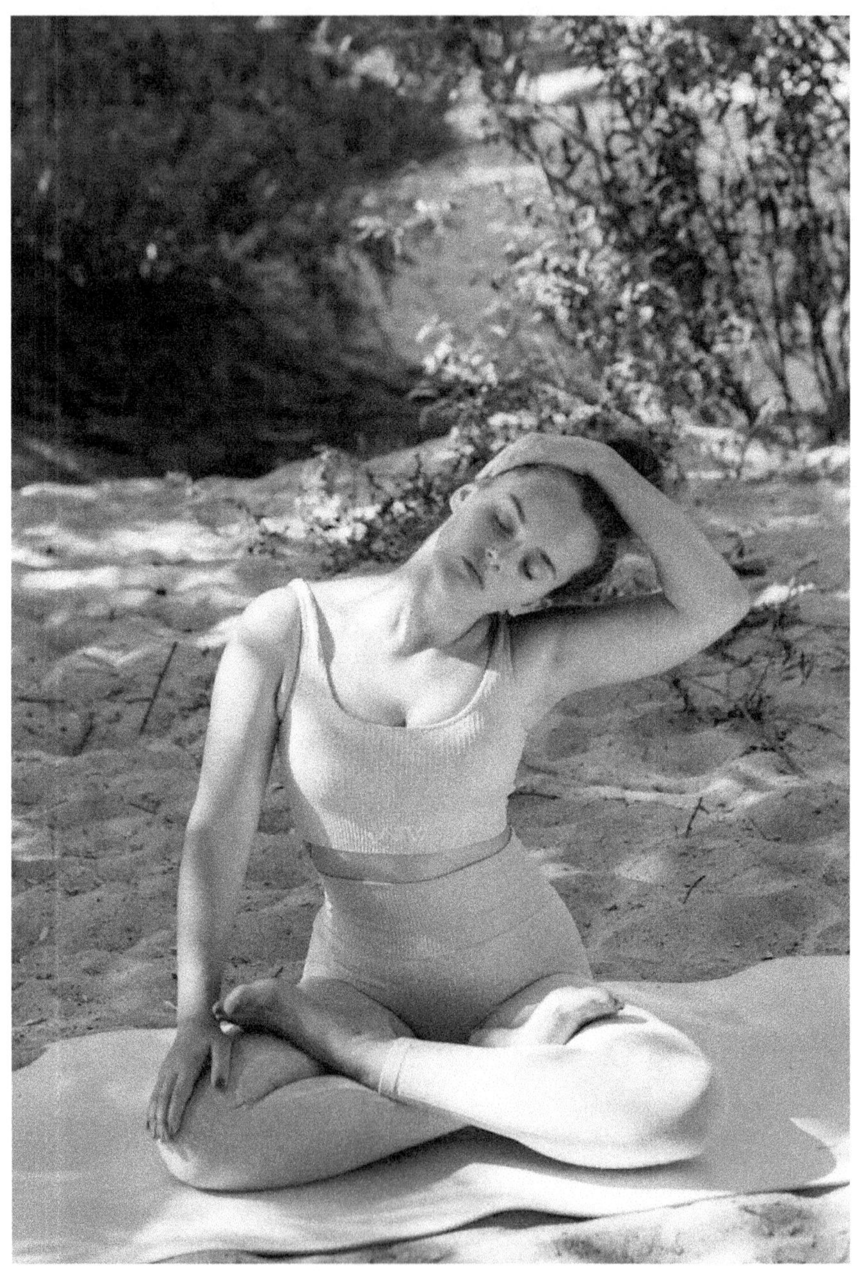

Seated Neck Release

LUNGING CALF STRETCH

This is a simple stretch that can be performed anywhere. Try using it when you have been waiting in a long line and need some relief for tired legs. This stretch is targeted for the calf muscles, but you can feel the benefits all the way up your leg and into your hip.

Begin this stretch with your hands on your hips. If you need added support, you can stand near and facing a wall so that you can reach out for extra balance.

- With your hands on your hips/wall step back with one foot.
- In a mini lunge position keep the back leg straight while pressing the heel of that foot towards the ground.
- Your front knee will be very slightly bent with the knee in line with your ankle.
- Do not extend the bent knee in front of your foot.
- Hold this stretch for 30 seconds and slowly bring the back leg back in line with the front.
- Switch sides and repeat.

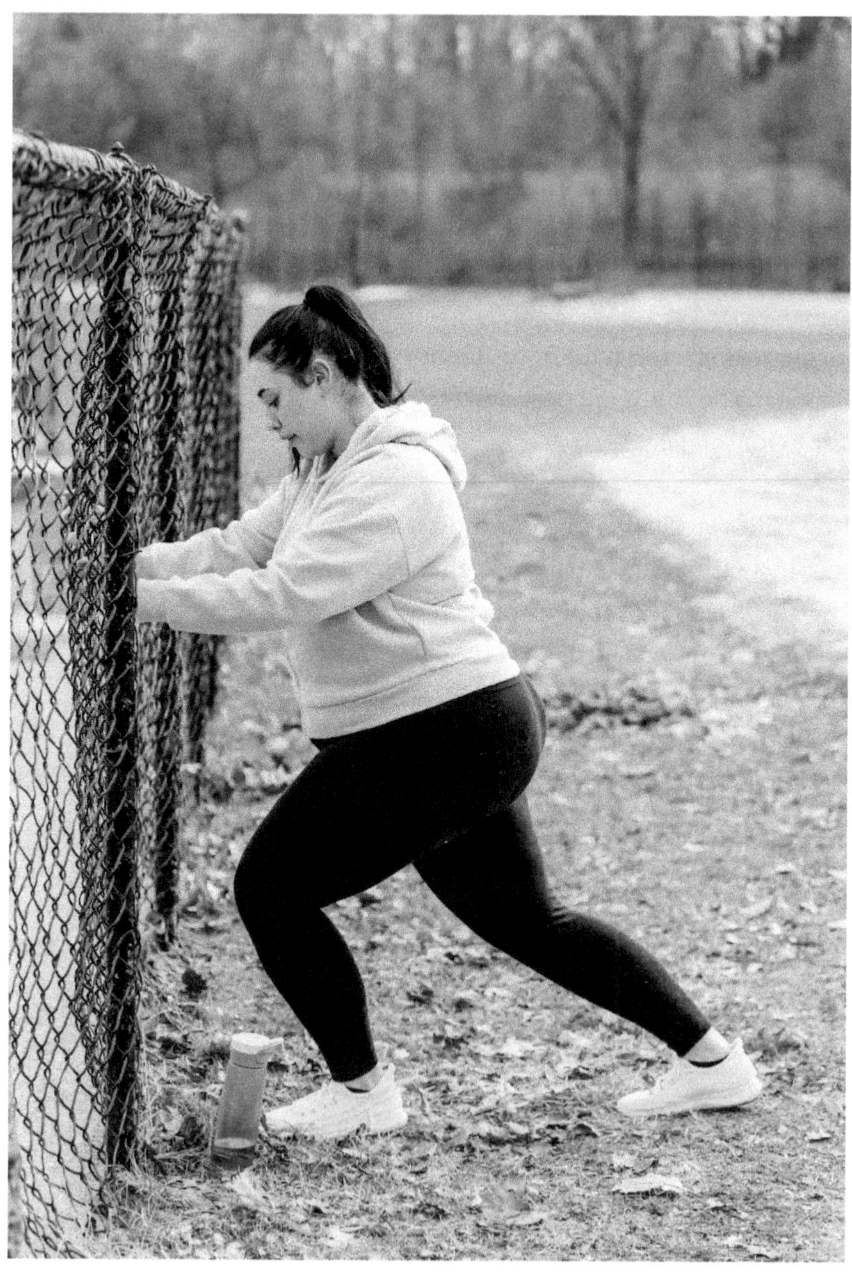

Lunging Calf Stretch

CROSS ARM STRETCH

The Cross Arm Stretch is wonderful for stretching the backs of your shoulders. For myself, when I do this stretch, I like to slowly lower my head to the shoulder opposite of the one that I am stretching. I like to relax into it and feel that it increases my stretch while adding benefit to my neck muscles. Again, this is a personal choice.

- Begin by reaching the arm to be stretched across your chest.
- Keeping the elbow straight, reach up with the opposite hand and place it on the straight arm at or right below the elbow.
- Pull the straight arm slowly across the body until the stretch is felt.
- Hold this stretch for 15-30 seconds.
- Switch arms and repeat the process.

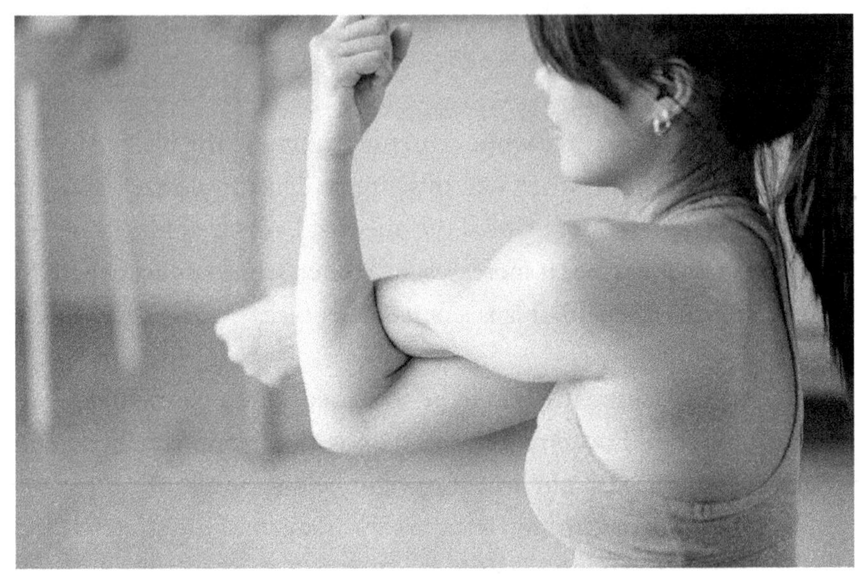

Cross Arm Stretch

TRICEP STRETCH

This stretch is for the muscle that runs down the back of your arm, the tricep. Repetitive movements such as long hours of typing can make this muscle tense. The tricep stretch can provide some much needed relief to this area.

- Begin this stretch by straightening one arm out in front of you.
- Turn your palm towards the sky and raise that arm high so that it is next to your ear.
- Next, bend your elbow as if you are going to touch your opposite shoulder or pat your own back.
- Looking straight ahead, take the opposite hand, grab your folded elbow and gently pull back until you can feel a stretch.
- Hold for 15-30 seconds, release and repeat the process with the opposite arm.

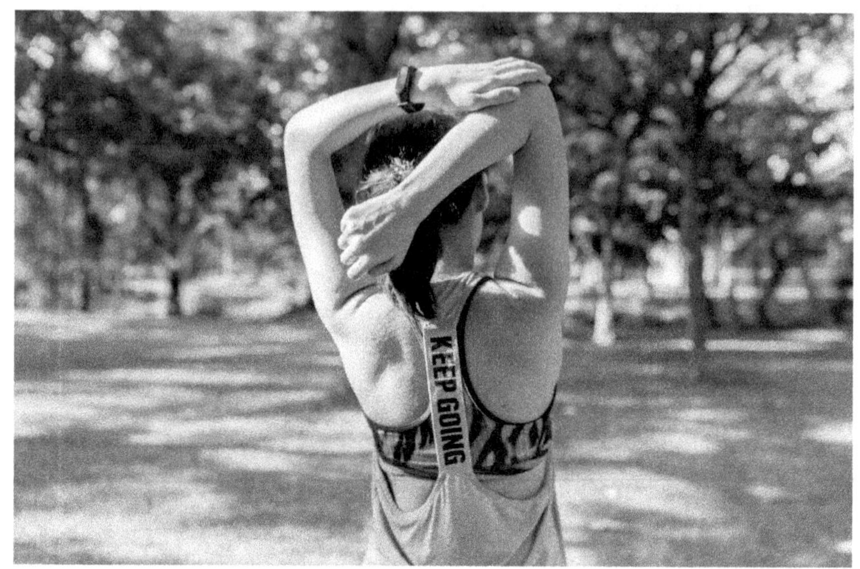

Tricep Stretch

SUPINE LEG STRETCH

This leg stretch is one that is good from your ankle all the way into your lower back. It helps to relieve muscle stress and tension from common everyday activities.

- Begin by laying on your back with both knees bent and looking up at the ceiling/sky.
- Slowly raise one leg keeping it straight.
- You can grab that calf muscle in your hands and gently pull, making sure to stop at a comfortable point where you can feel the stretch.
- Alternate between pointing and flexing your toes.
- Hold this stretch for 30 seconds as comfort and balance permits.
- Release and lower that leg back to the bent knee position.
- Repeat the process with the opposite leg.

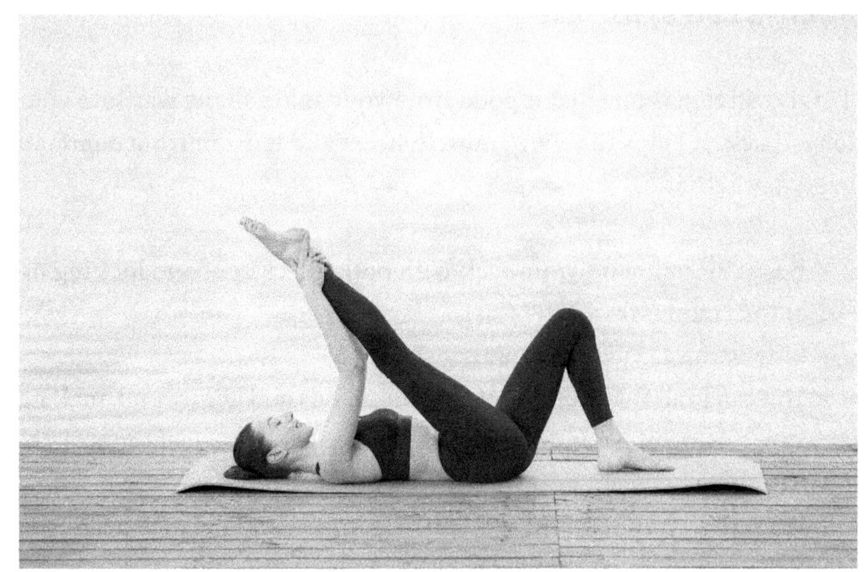

Supine Leg Stretch

STANDING QUAD STRETCH

The quadricep muscle is in the front upper thigh portion of your leg. These muscles are engaged often and when you are doing everyday tasks such as walking, running, squatting and lunging. The standing quad stretch is a nice stretch to give these muscles some much needed attention.

- As this stretch requires balance, you may want to stand beside a wall and place your hand there for added support.
- Begin with the outside foot (the one farthest from the wall) slowly lift your leg bending the knee back so that your foot is going towards your rear.
- Grab that foot in your hand and hold or gently pull back until you can feel the stretch in the front of your thigh.
- Hold for 15-30 seconds as comfortable, release your foot and lower it to the ground.
- Turn your body so that your opposite side is towards the wall and repeat the process with the other leg.

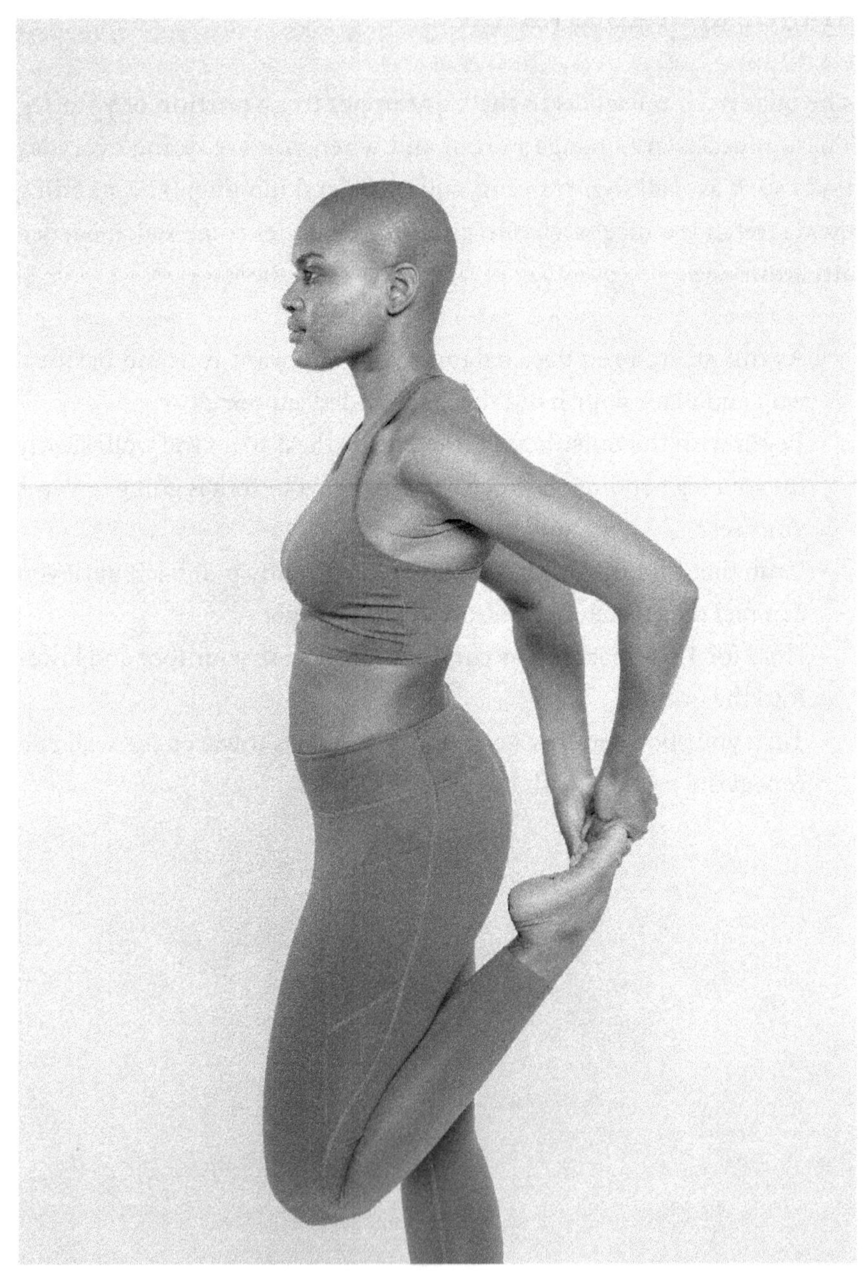

Standing Quad Stretch

HAPPY BABY STRETCH

The happy baby is considered a yoga pose and I love using this stretch to relieve tension in my lower back. Our lower backs take on a great amount of stress throughout the day whether we are standing or sitting. Our back muscles are involved in nearly everything that we do and deserve some much needed attention.

- Begin this stretch by laying on your back with knees bent.
- Slowly raise your feet bringing your knees towards your chest.
- Reach up with both hands to grab hold of the bottoms of your feet while letting your knees fall open and to the sides.
- If holding onto your feet poses a challenge, you can modify this stretch by holding your ankles or shins.
- Hold this position for 30-60 seconds as comfort allows.

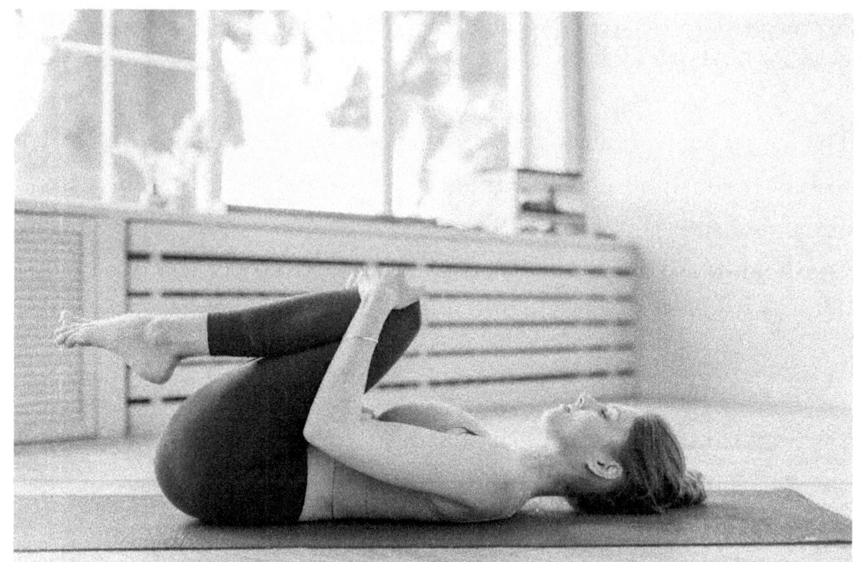

Happy Baby Stretch

BALANCE

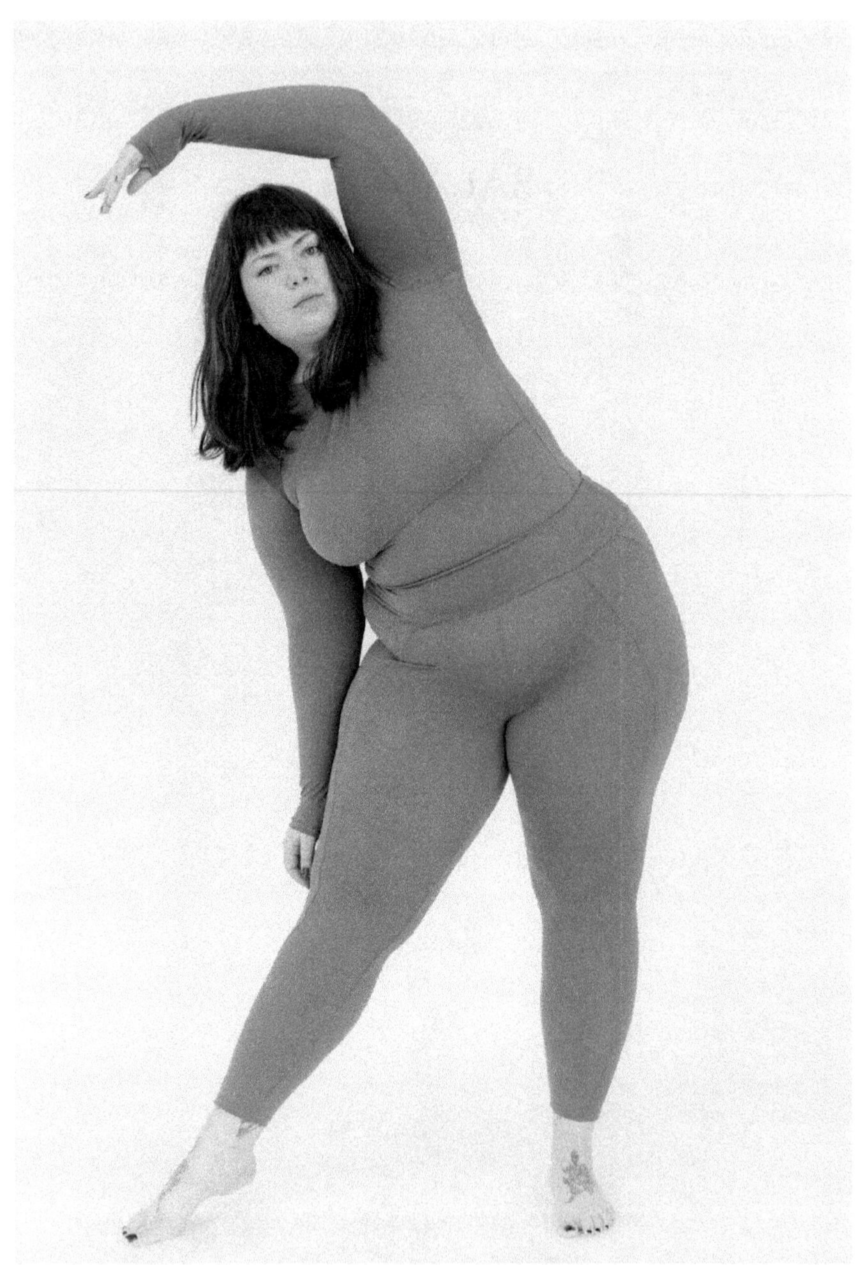

As stated previously, exercise is not exclusive to just one category. I find this especially true with the balance exercises that I will be sharing with you. When we are performing a balance exercise or pose, we are simultaneously strengthening a specific muscle or area of our body. Balance and strength training coexist and you will notice that being reflected in these two specific areas of this book.

Often with balance we are strengthening our core. Having a strong core is important and helps improve many aspects of our body and overall health. Building a strong core will improve your strength, balance and stability. It can also reduce back pain, and improve posture.

Some of the following exercises will focus on trunk and core activation with the goal being to help to create a more stable base when doing some of the standing moves.

Standing Balance

Building strong feet, ankles and calves can really improve your balance. Try doing this move slowly as it is also helping to build that strong core.

- Begin by standing with your spine straight and feet slightly parted
- Engage your core as you slowly raise up on your toes.
- Breathing through the pose, concentrate on maintaining posture, balance , and a strong core.
- Try holding for 15 seconds and lowering your feet back to the ground.
- Repeat this balance 10 times.

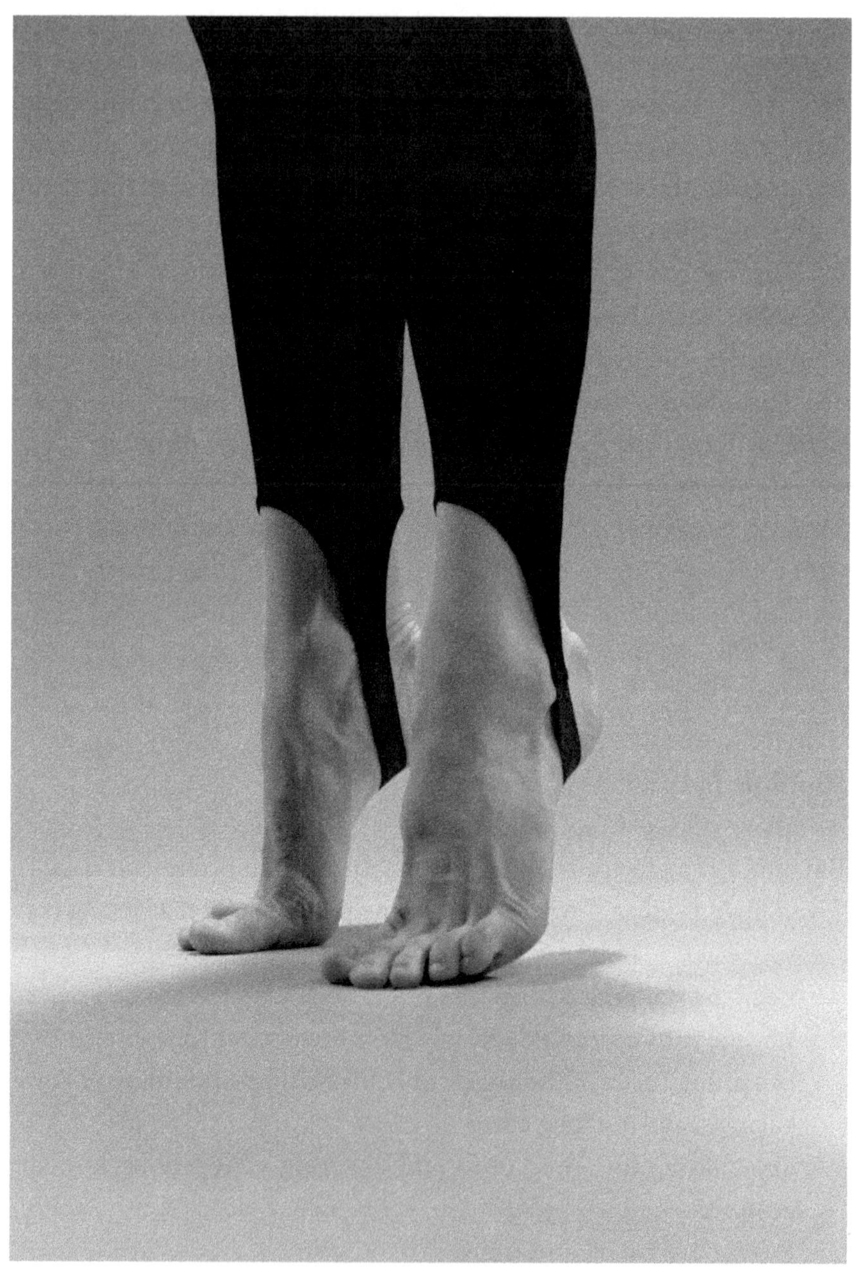

Standing Balance

PRONE HUNDRED

This is another exercise done laying on the floor or a mat. This core strengthening exercise will require you to balance your weight as you distribute it evenly between your abdomen and hips. You will be working to improve lower back strength and ultimately creating a stronger base of support.

- Begin this exercise by lying face down on the floor/mat.
- Bend your arms together in front of you and relax your forehead on your bent arms.
- With legs extended, raise upper and lower portions of your body until you have balanced and equally distributed your weight from your pelvic region to your ribs.
- Lengthen your spine and while breathing in for a five count, clap your feet together.
- Do the same as you release your breath out for a five count.
- Try doing this repetition 10 times to reach a count of 100.

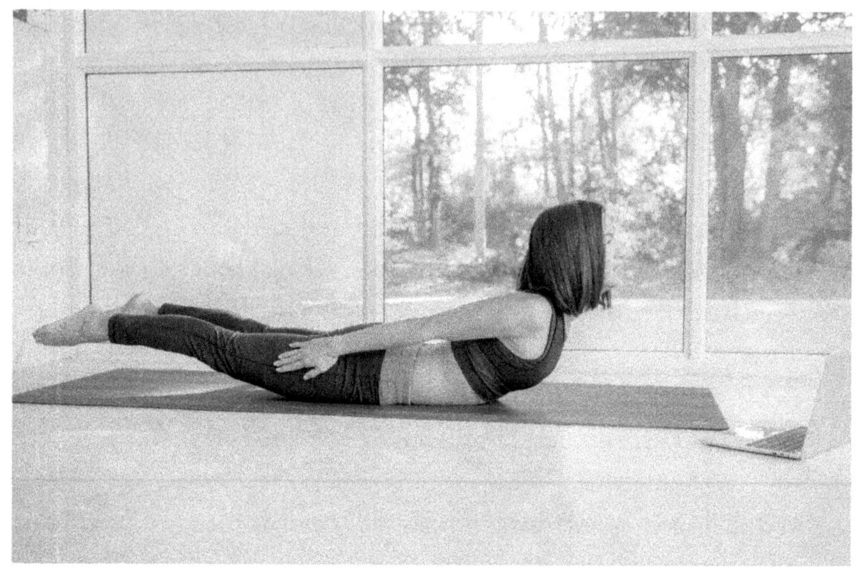

Prone Hundred

CORKSCREW

The corkscrew is another exercise done by laying on the floor or a mat. It is also an exercise where balancing your shifting body weight will help to strengthen the core and back muscles while also engaging your hip flexors.

- Begin by laying on your back with your legs straight.
- Placing your arms either by your sides, stretched out in a T position, or folded beneath your head, slowly raise your legs straight up keeping them together.
- Your lifted legs will begin in the twelve o'clock position and then you will engage your core muscles as you rotate them in a clockwise manner.
- Maintain balance as you rotate your legs in a circle before returning them to the twelve o'clock position.
- This will look like: legs in the air in front of you, lower them as you rotate them to the left, bring them forward straight out, and rotate to the right before bringing them straight up at the starting position.
- Make sure to maintain balance and keep your legs lifted off of the floor throughout the whole rotation.
- Finally, repeat the steps going in the opposite direction to complete one full set. Try repeating the set three times.

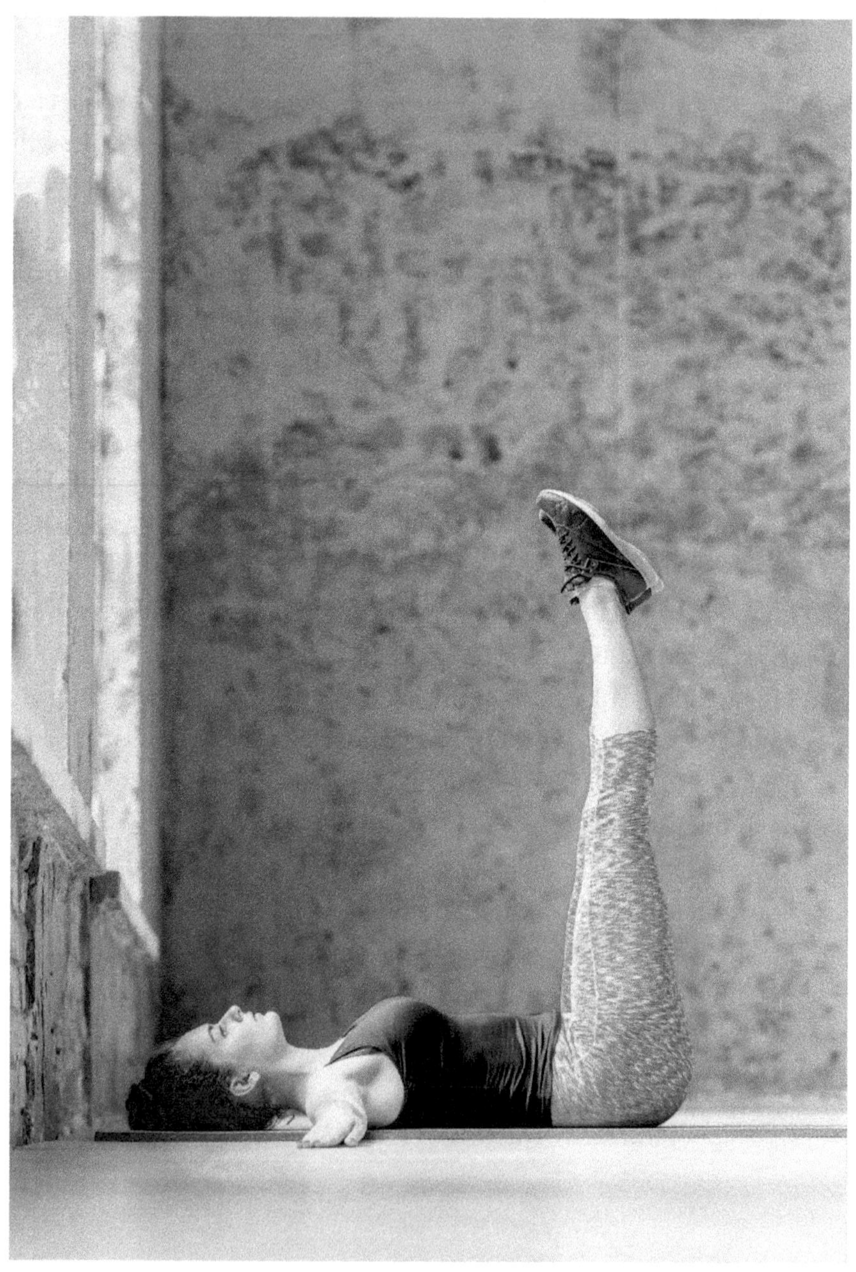

Corkscrew

TREE POSE

The tree pose is a good exercise for so many things, some of which include helping balance and posture while strengthening your legs and providing sciatic relief. This pose can also be beneficial to stress and concentration as you breathe through the exercise and work to maintain your form. Beginners may want to look for modifications to this pose. Some ideas could be to stand beside a wall and use a hand for support as you gain better balance. You could also try by starting with your foot perched lower on your leg.

- Begin by standing tall with your feet forward facing and slightly apart.
- Stretch your arms above your head elongating your spine.
- Engage your core to help with balance as you raise your right foot to perch on the inner thigh of your left leg.
- Keep your hips straight and avoid rotating them.
- You can move your hands to rest on your hips to help with balance.
- Breathe through the pose focusing on balance and control.
- Try holding this pose for 15-30 seconds.
- Lower your foot back to the starting position and repeat with the other side.

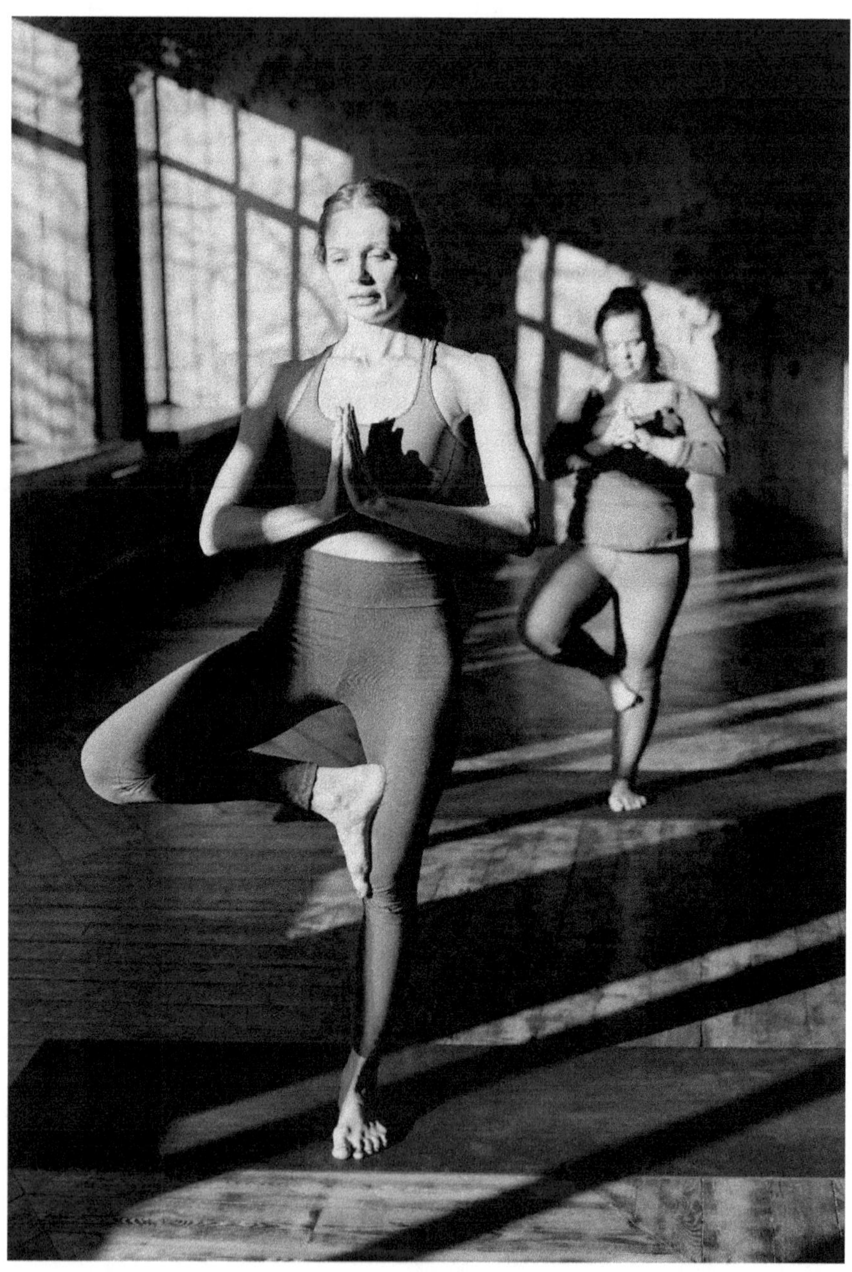

Tree Pose

BIRD DOG

The Bird Dog is another exercise that is good for targeting your core, while also strengthening your hips and back muscles. The balance required for this movement helps work on your posture and overall mobility

- Begin the exercise on all fours with your shoulders and knees aligned.
- Your hands will be placed directly under and in line with your shoulders, while your knees will be directly in line with and under your hips.
- Maintain a straight spine in the neutral position. Do not arch or sag.
- With your head down and in line with your spine, raise your right arm and left leg, extending each into the straight position.
- Make sure that you do not raise your leg so high that your spine loses alignment. Nore should your hips rotate.
- After holding this position for a few seconds, lower your extremities back to the floor and repeat with the opposite side.
- Try doing 3 sets of ten repetitions.

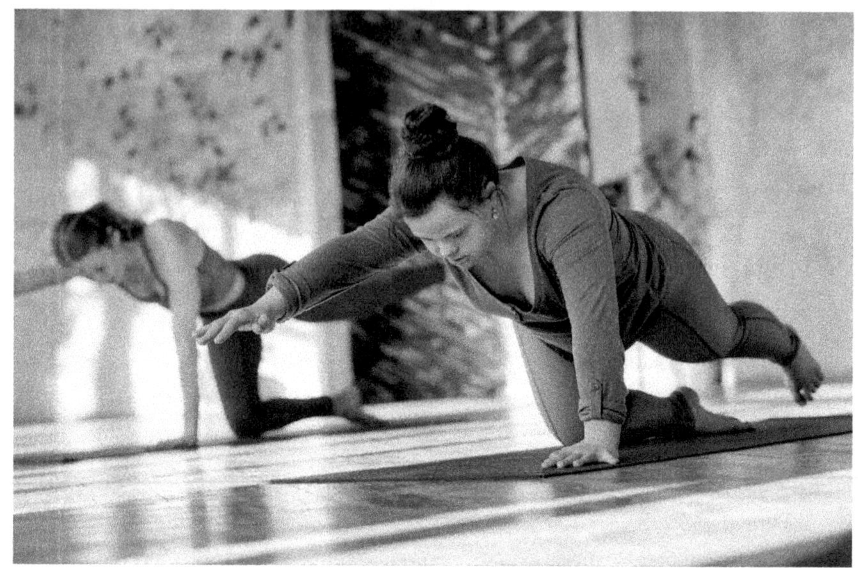

Bird Dog

Rotational Push-up

The rotational push-up focuses on building strength in multiple muscles while integrating natural movements of pushing, pulling, and rotating. Stabilization of muscle groups and balance play a key role in this movement.

- Begin face down in a push-up or high plank position with your hands and toes on the ground, arms straight and legs extended behind you.
- With arms shoulder width apart and hands directly below your shoulders, perform a push-up by bending your elbows to lower your torso as close to the ground as possible without touching.
- Push your body back up to the starting position and begin rotating your trunk while reaching towards the ceiling with one arm. Your heels will come together and rotate down towards the floor as you do this.
- Hold at the top of this position for a couple of seconds and rotate so that your body is back in line and return to the starting position.
- Repeat the process and rotate to the opposite side after your next push-up. A completion of the movements on both sides is one repetition . Try doing 10 of these repetitions.
- If this is too challenging in the beginning, remove the push-up step and just do the body rotations holding the pose at the top.

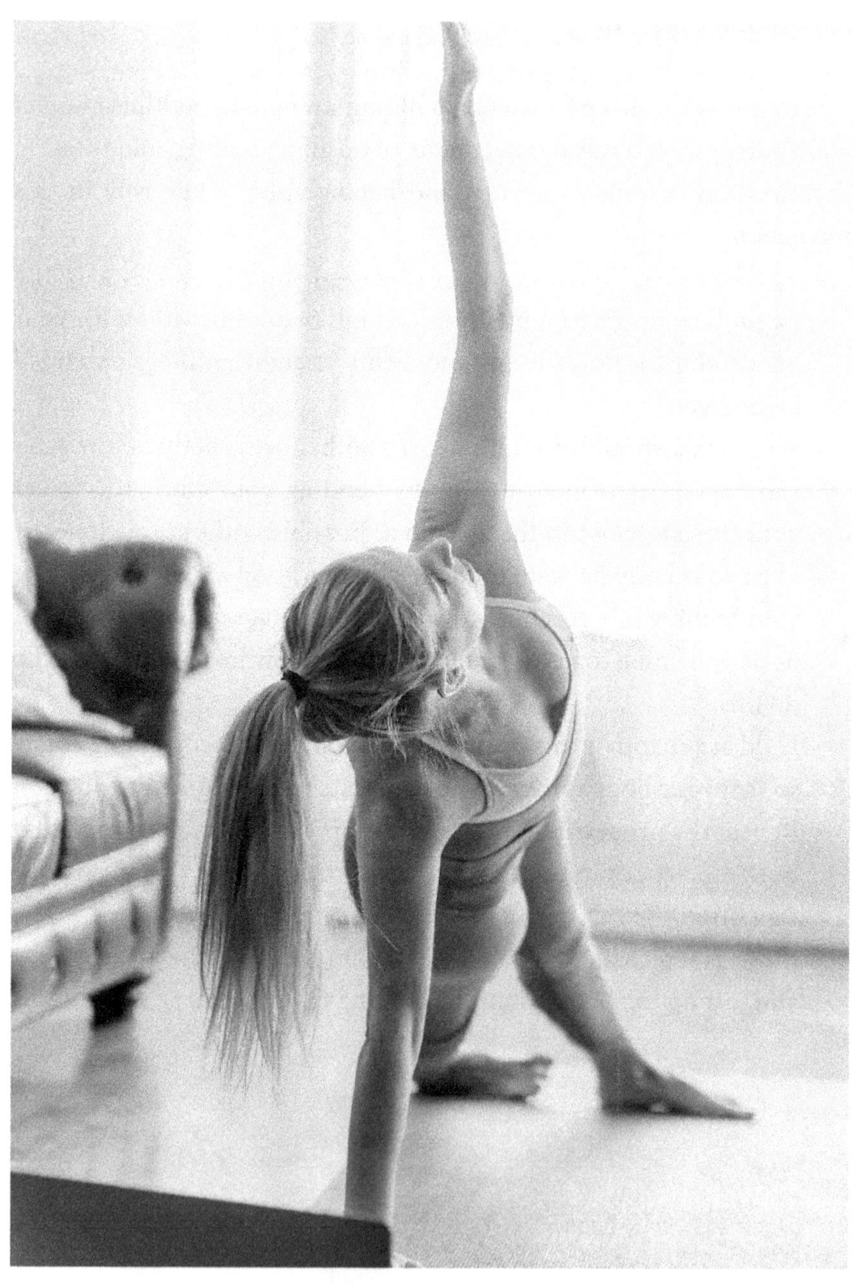

Rotational Push-up

BALANCE

37

STRENGTH

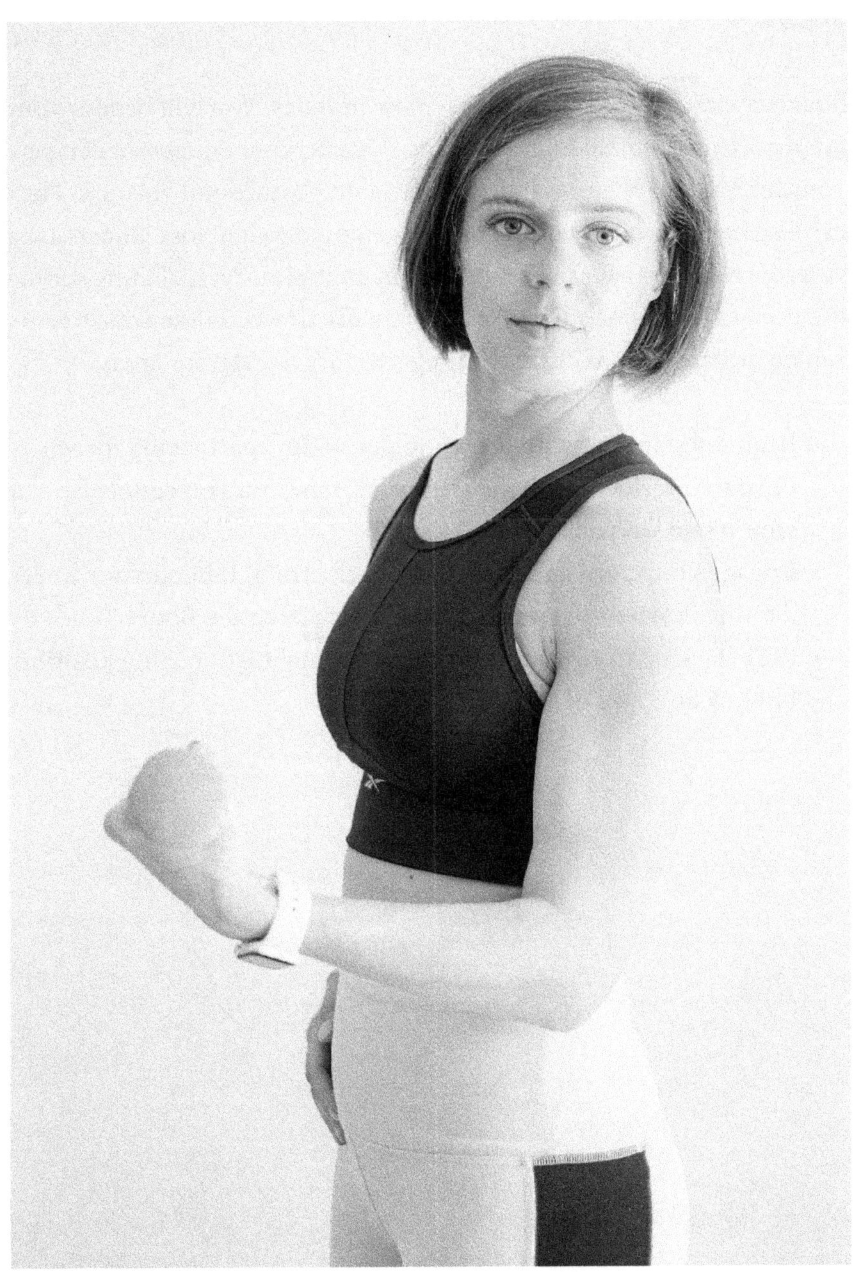

SQUATS

Squats are an exercise that works many muscles. You will benefit your quadricep and gluteal muscles using this exercise. Squats also engage your hips and core and can be beneficial to posture and balance. They can also help you burn calories and possibly aid weight loss. Squats are a versatile exercise that can be modified in multiple ways including adding the use of weights or adjusting how you dip down. These adjustments can be utilized to maximize training and target different areas.

- Begin by standing with feet shoulder width apart facing forward.
- I like to interlock my hands in front of me, but you could also put your hands on your head.
- Engage your core and with your back straight, bend your knees dipping down until your thighs are parallel to the floor.
- Push back up until you return to the straight leg starting position.
- I like to do 3 sets of 10 squats.

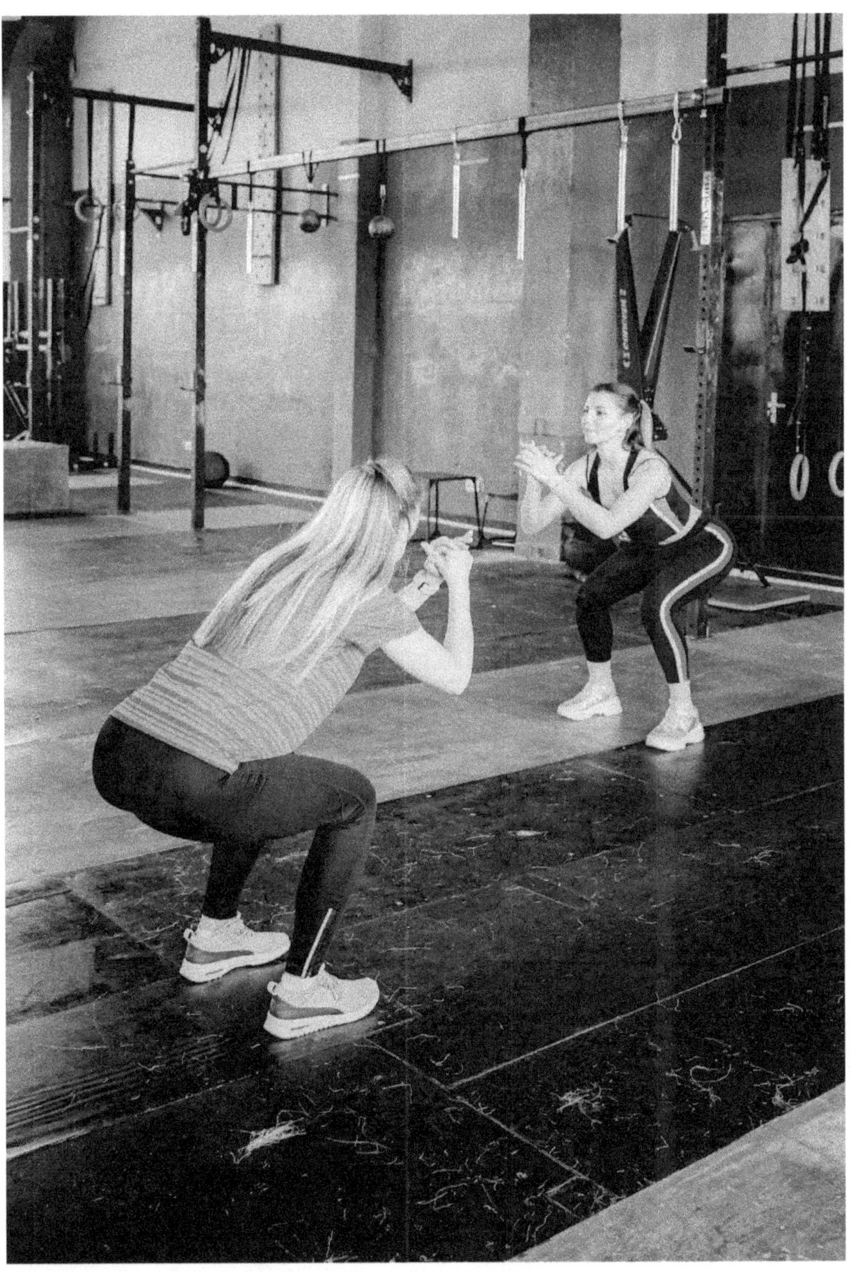

Squat

FROG SQUAT

To modify the traditional squat, try the frog squat.

- Again, start facing forward with feet shoulder width apart.
- Flex hips bending slightly forward with a minor bend to the knees.
- Rest your elbows on the insides of your knees.
- Keeping the elbows on your knees dip into a low/deep squat.
- Straightening the legs, push back up into a standing position.
- Repeat the steps doing 3 sets of 10.

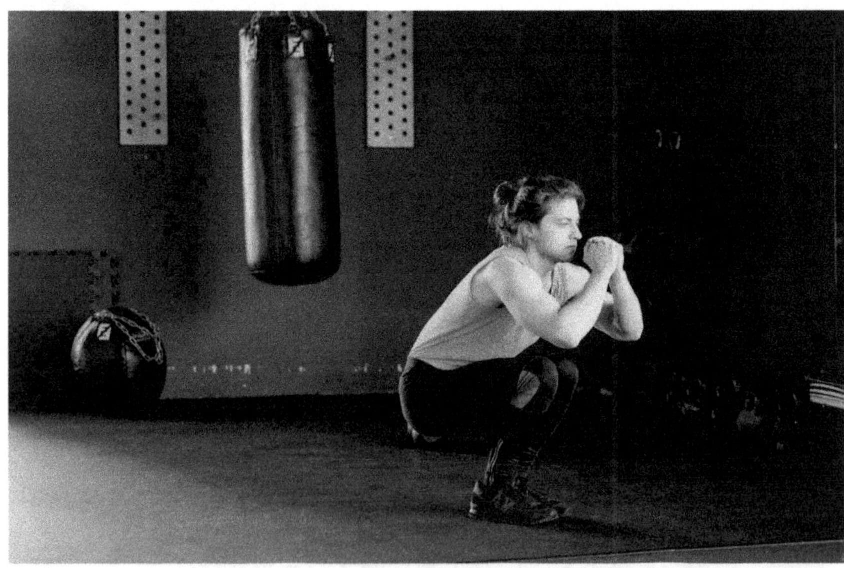

Frog Squat

PLANKS

Planks are an exercise that can be modified and performed in various ways. Planks are a great stand alone exercise and can also be incorporated into several others. Planks help improve your posture. They also help to strengthen muscles in your abs, back, neck, and shoulders. I like to perform a traditional low plank from my elbows.

- Begin laying face down on the floor/mat.
- For a low plank, lift up onto your elbows keeping them shoulder width apart.
- Raising your torso off the ground so that you are now on the balls of your feet and your elbows.
- Maintain a straight spine as you squeeze the abdominal muscles to engage the core.
- Breathing through this pose, see if you can hold this position for a full minute.

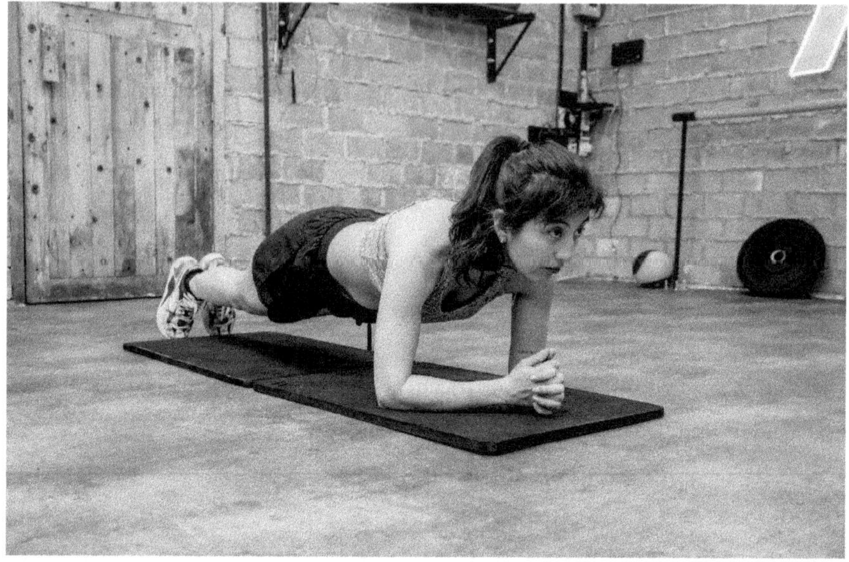

Plank

GLUTE/HAMSTRING BRIDGE

The Glute Bridge has many variations and is good for working your hips, abs, gluteus and hamstring muscles.

- For the basic Glute Bridge, begin by laying on your back with knees bent and feet flat on the ground about hip width apart.
- Keeping your shoulders on the floor/mat and arms at your sides or over your chest, push through your feet to raise your hips off the ground until they make a straight line with your shoulders.
- While breathing, hold this pose for a beat and then lower your hips back to the ground.
- I try to do 3 sets of 10.

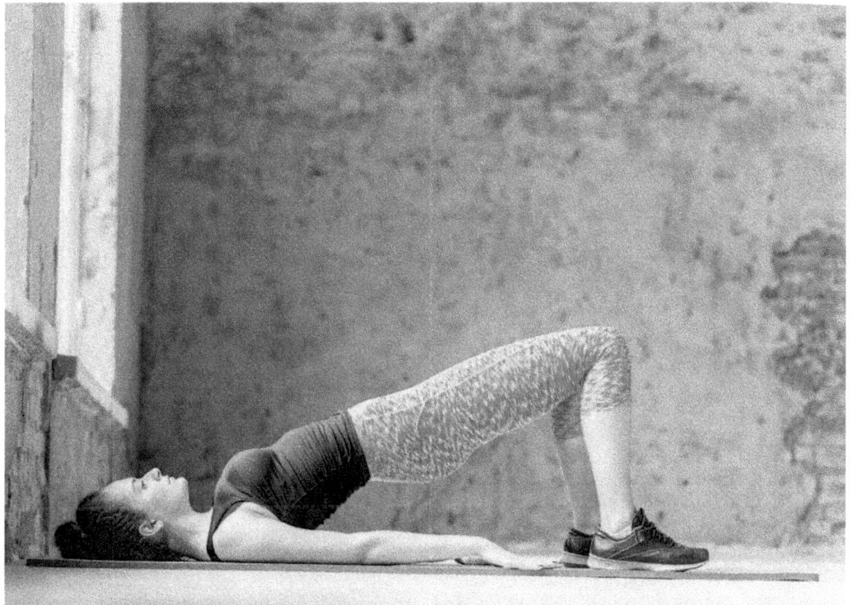

Glute/Hamstring Bridge

If you would like to challenge yourself on the Glute Bridge, alternate between legs, raising one straight up as you are in your bridge pose, then lower that leg and do the other. Try 10 of these.

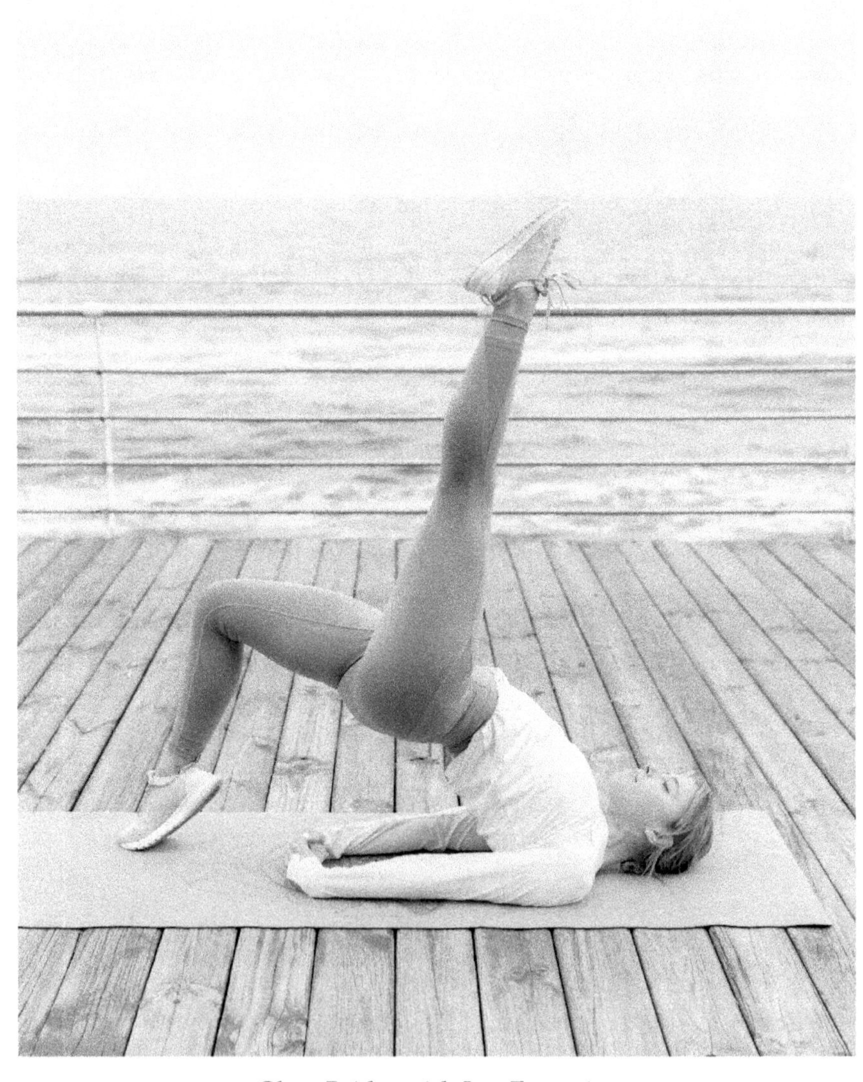

Glute Bridge with Leg Extension

FIRE HYDRANT

This exercise works the gluteus maximus. I love this exercise for lifting and shaping this aging bum. You can add a resistance band for additional difficulty.

- Begin this exercise on all fours. Hands should be on the floor/mat shoulder width apart, and your bent knees should be hip width apart in line with your hands.
- Keeping the spine straight, begin to raise one bent knee up towards the ceiling out to your side.
- Lower the knee back to the starting position.
- Do 10 of these on one side before switching legs and repeating the process. I like to do 3 sets of 10.

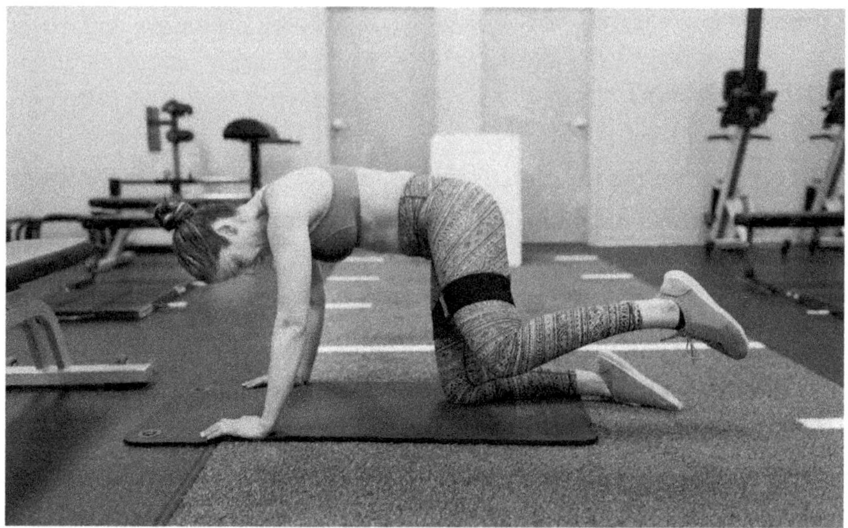

Fire Hydrant with Resistance Band

DONKEY KICK

This exercise is another favorite of mine for lifting and shaping my rear. I typically do this in conjunction with the fire hydrant switching between the two when doing my reps. For example, 10 fire hydrant lifts on the right leg, 10 donkey kicks on the same leg and then switch sides. This is just my personal preference.

- Begin this exercise on all fours. Hands should be on the floor/mat shoulder width apart, and your bent knees should be hip width apart in line with your hands.
- Keeping the spine straight, begin to raise one bent knee up and back, keeping the knee bent at 90 degrees as you simulate a kick behind you.

- Your leg should be parallel to the floor with your foot to the ceiling.
- Keeping your core engaged, hold this for a breath and lower your leg back to the floor. Try to do 10 of these and repeat that set 3 times.

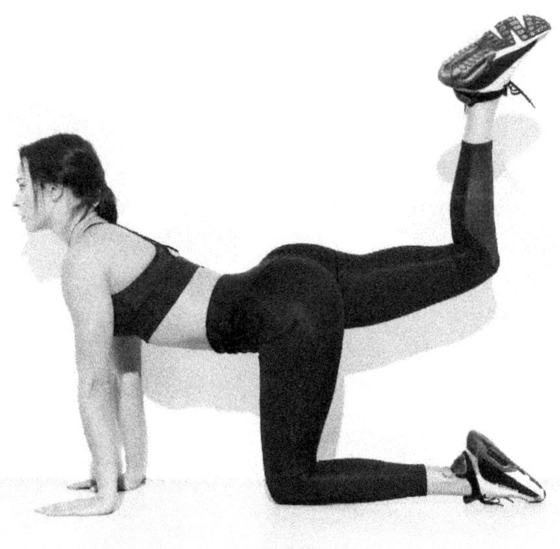

Donkey Kick

DUMBBELLS

There are so many easy at home exercises that can be done with a set of light weight dumbbells. I have recently purchased a set of adjustable dumbbells which allow you to drop or add weight to the same dumbbell depending on your needs or level of advancement. They are versatile and a space saver.

When I get the dumbbells out, I do a series of exercises from the same stance including, bicep curls, front raises, lateral side raises, and tricep extensions. I use 5 lb weights to begin with the option to increase or lessen weight as needed. Since my goal is toning and not building large muscles I tend to stick with less weight.

BICEP CURL

- Begin with feet shoulder width apart, spine straight with shoulders back and knees slightly bent.
- You should have a dumbbell in each hand by your side with your palms facing out.
- Tighten your stomach muscles to engage your core as you slowly raise the dumbbells towards your shoulders. I like to do both at the same time, but you can alternate arms if you choose. Just make sure to do the same number of reps for each arm.
- The movement is coming from your elbows bending. Do not shrug your shoulders.
- After reaching a full flex and completing the curl, lower the weights with palms facing up, and repeat the move.
- I like to do 10 before switching to the next move.

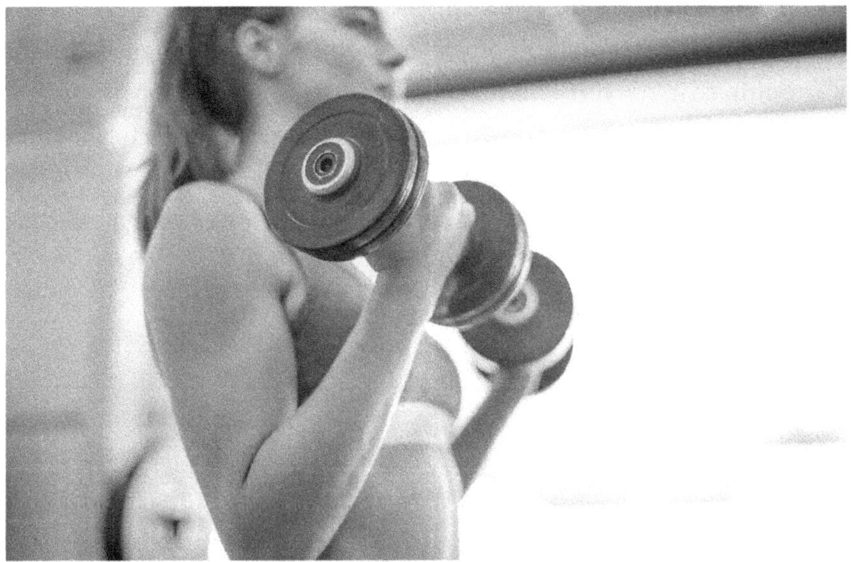

Bicep Curl

FRONT RAISES

- Using the same stance, turn your hands over so that your palms are

facing down towards your thighs.
- Again, engage your core muscles as you raise the weights straight out in front of you.
- Your palms are facing down as you raise the dumbbells to shoulder height.
- Keeping the stomach tight and arms straight, lower your arms back to the starting position.
- Repeat 10 times.

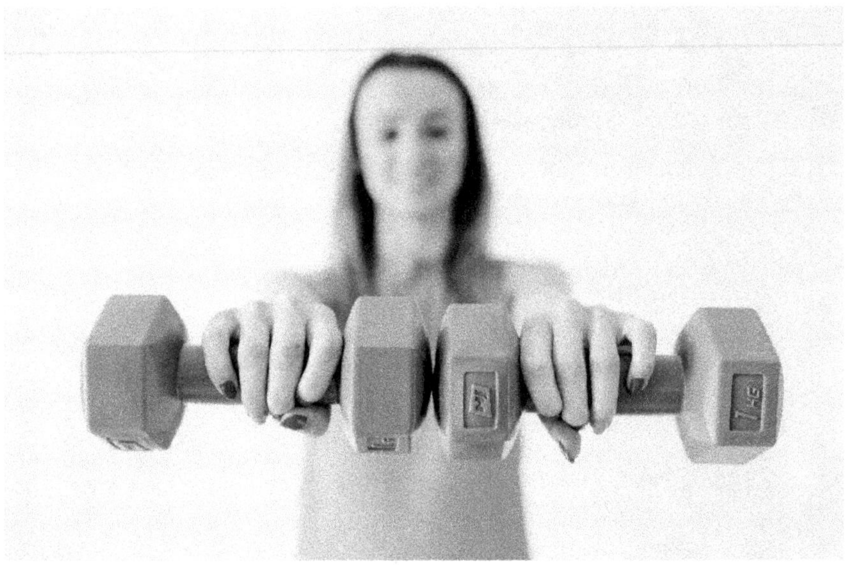

Front Raises

LATERAL SIDE RAISES

- Using the same stance again, bring the dumbbells to hang by your sides with your palms facing in towards your outer thighs.
- Engaging your core muscles and keeping your arms straight , raise them up at your sides until they are shoulder height.
- Keeping your back straight and your core engaged, lower your arms back to your sides.
- Repeat 10 times.

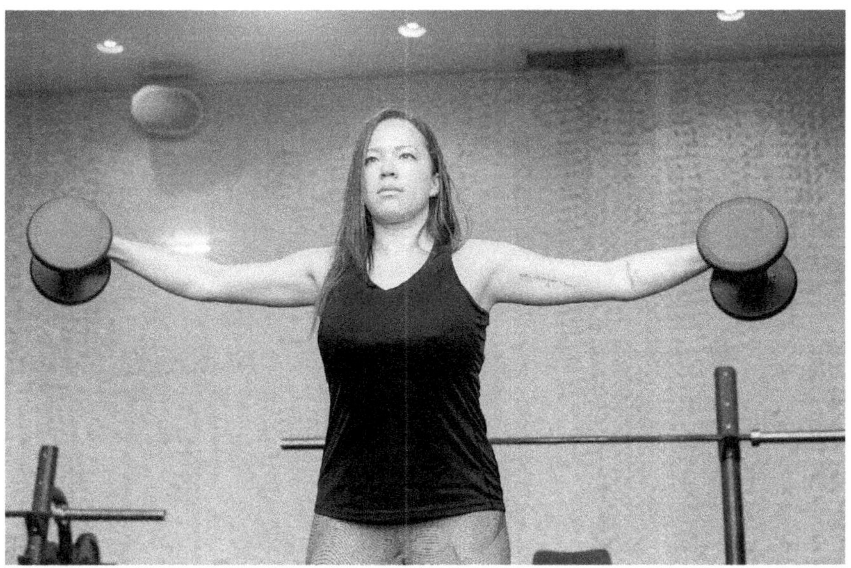

Lateral Side Raises

TRICEP EXTENSION

- Again using the same stance, you are just changing your grip on the dumbbells. This exercise can be done holding one dumbbell in both hands, or using both dumbbells in individual hands.
- Raise the dumbbells directly over your head with your palms facing each other and arms fully extended.
- Keeping the spine straight and core engaged, bend your elbows so that you are lowering the weights behind your head.
- Once you reach a full bend of the elbow, reverse the motion pushing the weights back over your head until your arms are again fully extended. Repeat 10 times.

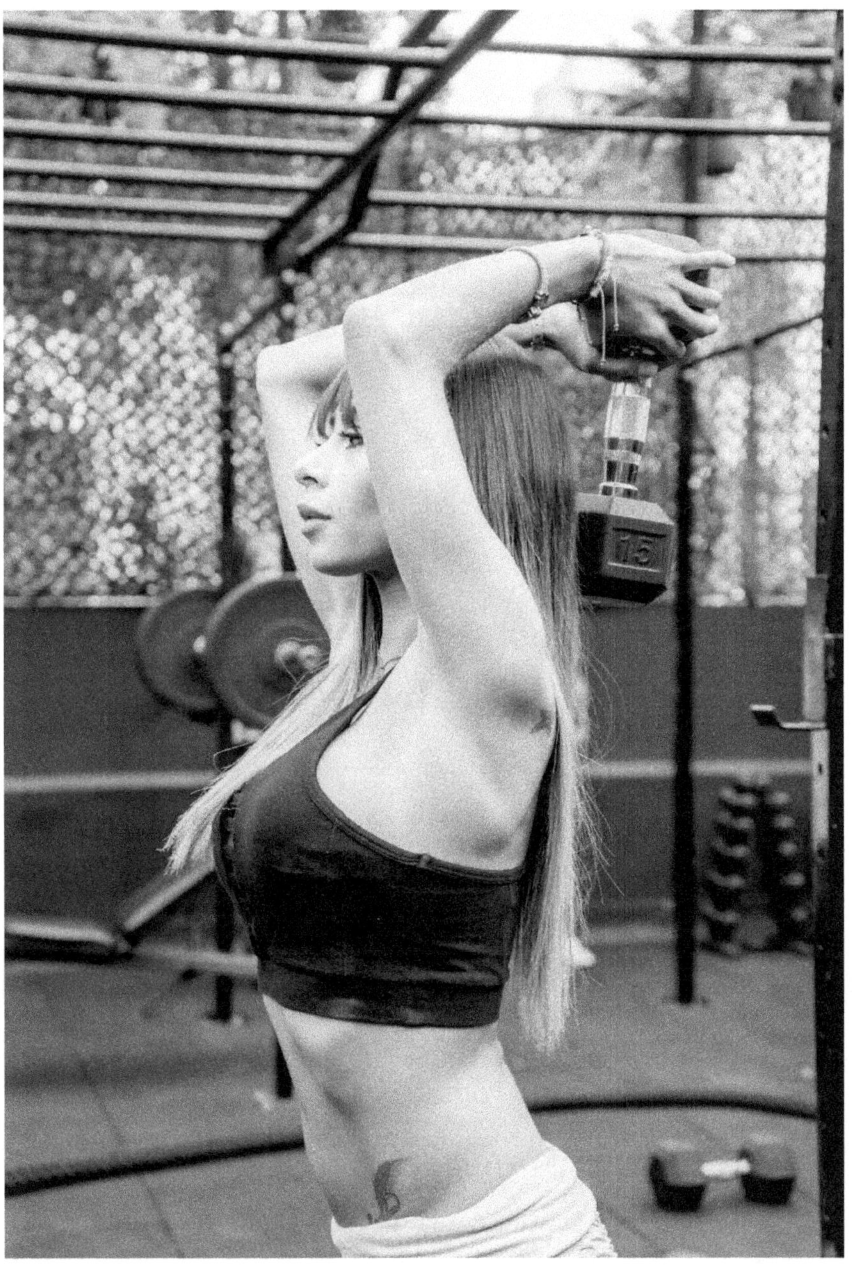

Tricep Extension

56

57

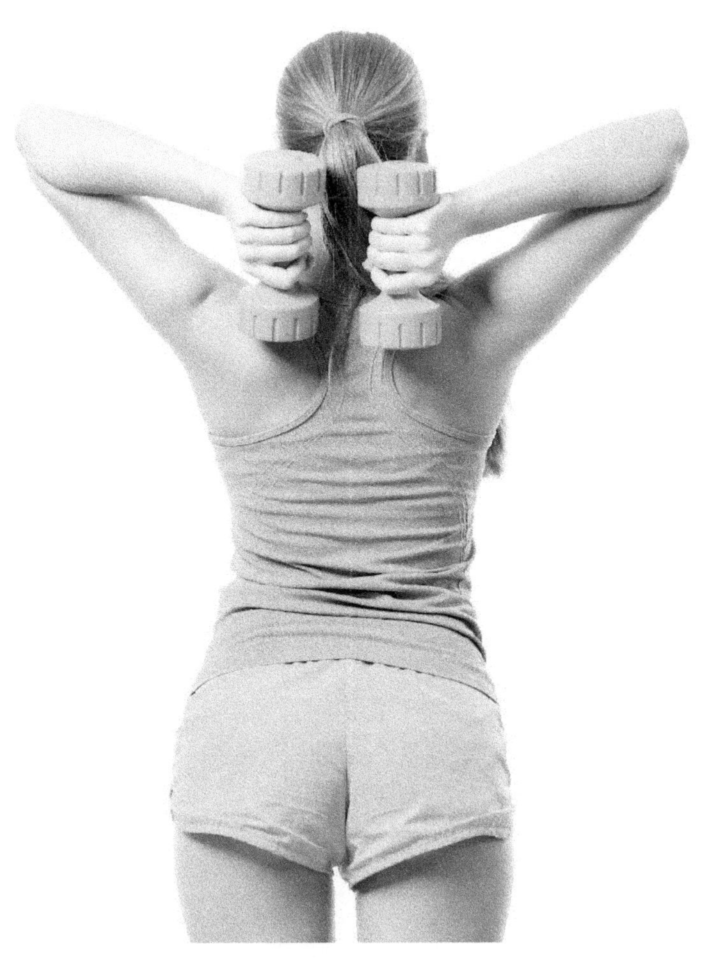

Tricep Extension

AEROBIC

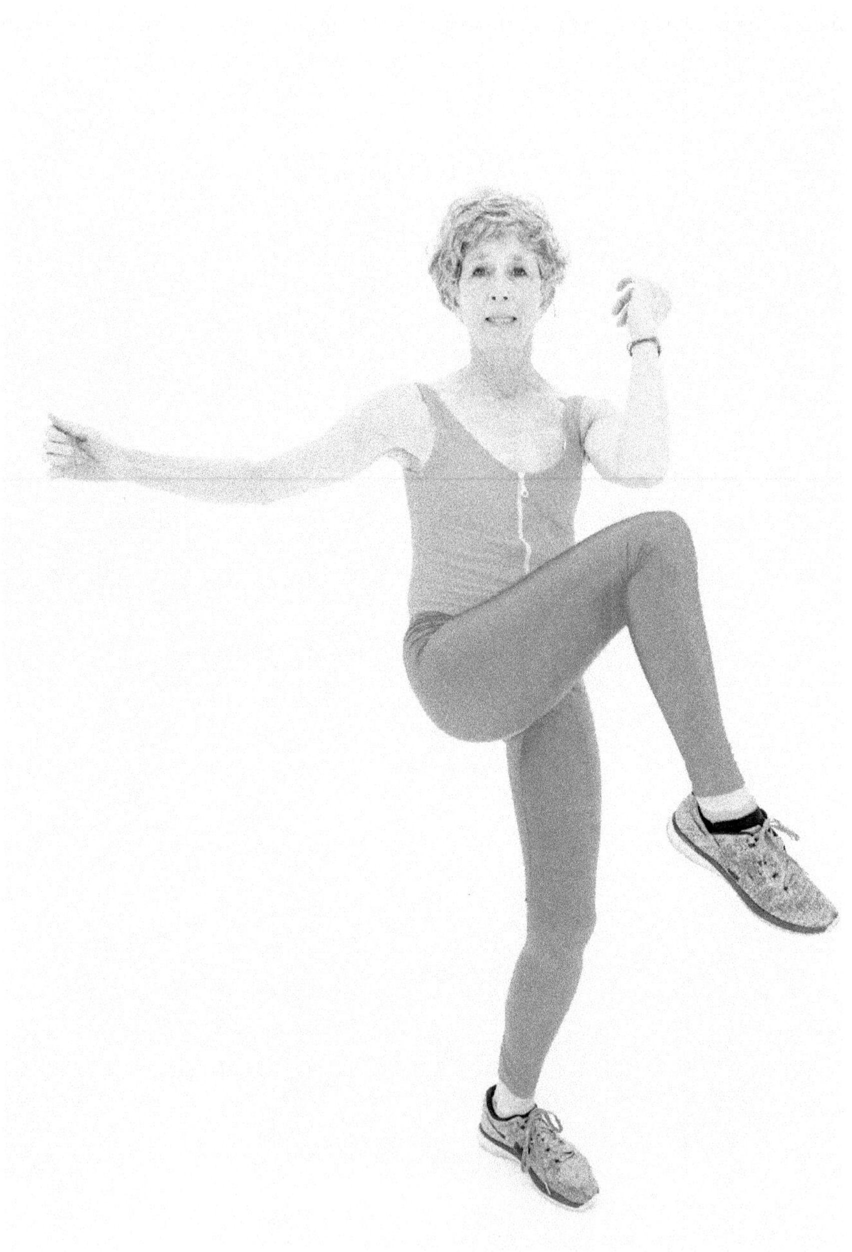

Aerobic exercise is probably the style of exercise that I do the least amount of at home. However, I do fit it in throughout my day by walking as much and whenever I can. I also have a semi recumbent bike at home that I will pull in front of the TV so that I can enjoy a show while I ride for twenty to thirty minutes. Having said that, there are many aerobic exercises that you can do from your living room requiring little to no equipment.

Dancing is a particular favorite of mine. I dance often, and it does not have to be structured dance. Turn some music on and cut loose. My house cleaning easily turns into anaerobic workout for me when I turn my favorite playlist on. There are also several wonderful dance based workouts that can be found online if you prefer to follow a guided lesson.

Other aerobic activities that I enjoy include swimming, jogging, and using an elliptical. However, I can not do these exercises while inside my home. There are many parks, trails, and neighborhoods near me that make great places to take myself away for a jog. Most of my swimming and elliptical riding are done when I am on the road traveling as I have access to a pool and weight room then.

As mentioned previously, exercise crosses platforms and is not exclusive to one category. Many of the exercises mentioned in this book are already giving you a cardio workout. While Aerobic exercise is not my go to during my time at home, I am actually getting a cardiovascular workout while I perform some of my other favorite exercises. It is important to find movements that will increase your heart rate for an extended time and many of the exercises that I have already included will actually do this, but I have included some that are more specifically categorized as aerobic.

JUMP ROPE

Jumping rope is a great way to elevate your heart rate. It can be a stand alone exercise or be included in a circuit of other exercises to create a complete cardio workout. To create a circuit, choose an exercise to perform for 30-60 seconds, then rest for 20 seconds and move on to another exercise. I like to do this with about five exercises and then start over with the first. I do this for about ten minutes, or 3-4 full circuits.

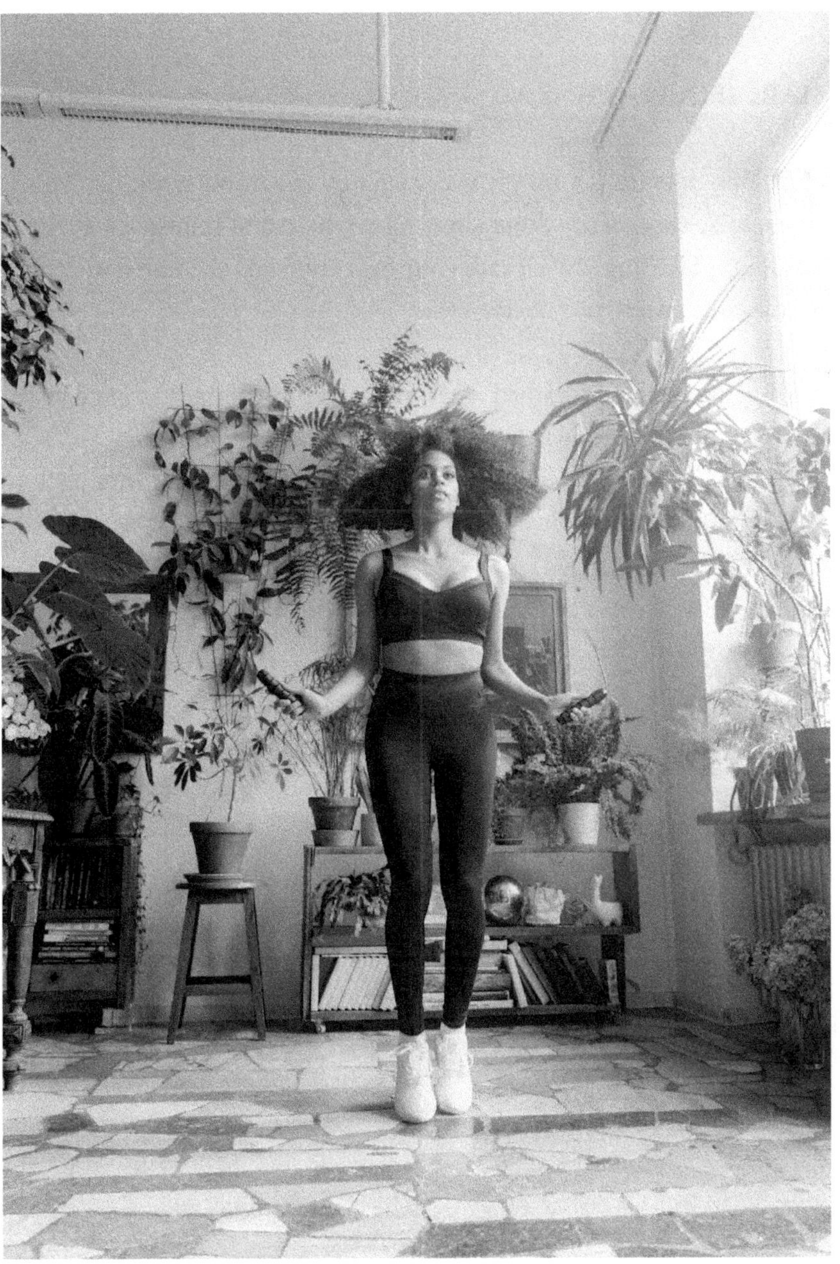

Jump Rope

MARCH IN PLACE

Marching in place is a simple way to get in an aerobic workout. This is an exercise that can be done almost anywhere and requires no special training. Marching will elevate your heart rate and the intensity can be modified to meet your needs.

- Begin by facing forward with feet at a comfortable distance apart.
- The march is done by alternating between legs.
- Bend one knee up towards your chest, lowering that foot back to the ground and doing the same with the other.

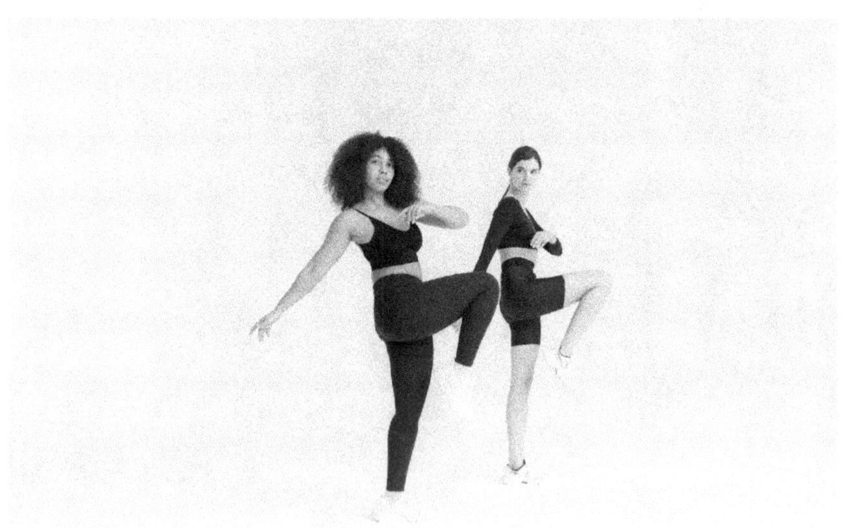

March In Place

HIGH KNEES

One way to increase the intensity of marching in place is by turning your march into a high knees exercise.

- To do this simply increase the speed and rate at which you raise your knees.
- Turn a standard march into almost a jog, where you raise your knees up higher towards your chest and at a faster rate of speed.

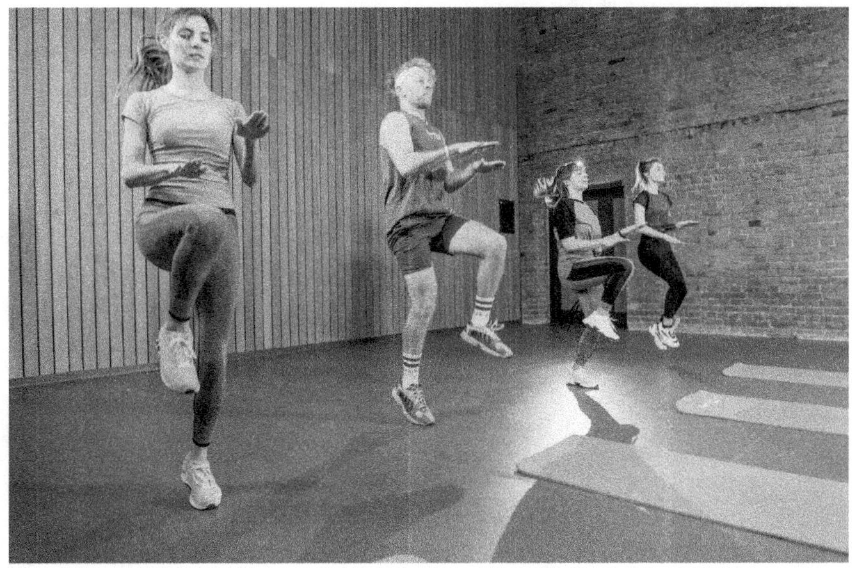

High Knees

KNEES TO ELBOWS

Knees to elbow is an aerobic exercise that can help enhance mobility. This exercise can work your core and hip flexors while also giving you a cardio workout.

- Begin in a standing position with your feet facing forward about shoulder width apart.
- You can perform this exercise with your arms bent at chest level, or challenge yourself and raise your bent arms up, placing your hands on the back of your head.
- With your arms in either position raise one knee towards your chest while simultaneously rotating your hips so that your opposite elbow touches that knee.
- After the elbow touch, lower that leg back to the ground and do the same movement to the opposite side. Alternate sides for the duration of this exercise for your chosen amount of time.

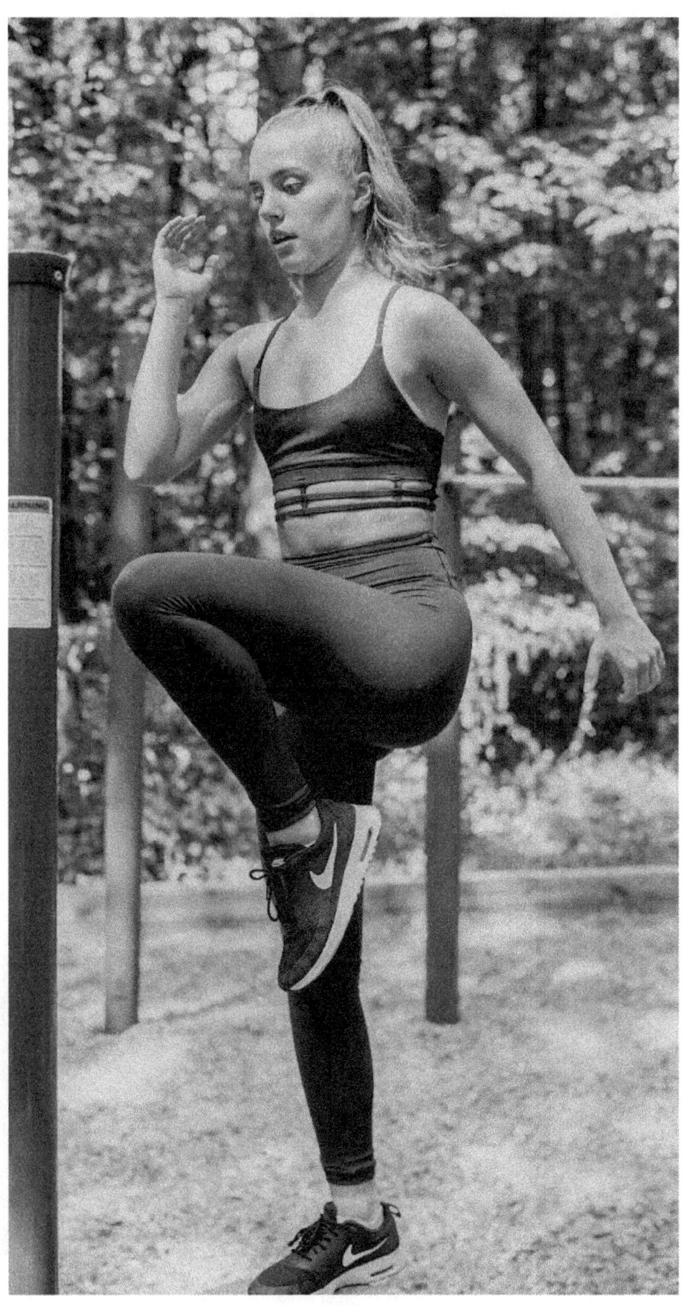

Knees to Elbows

ARM CIRCLES

Arm circles can be done both from a standing and sitting position. I prefer to do these while standing.

- Stand with your feet facing forward about shoulder width apart.
- Keep your back straight, engage your abs and extend both arms straight out to your sides.
- You will proceed by making a forward circular motion with your arms in this position. After a ten count in the forward motion, you can reverse the movement so that you are doing the arm circles in the opposite direction.

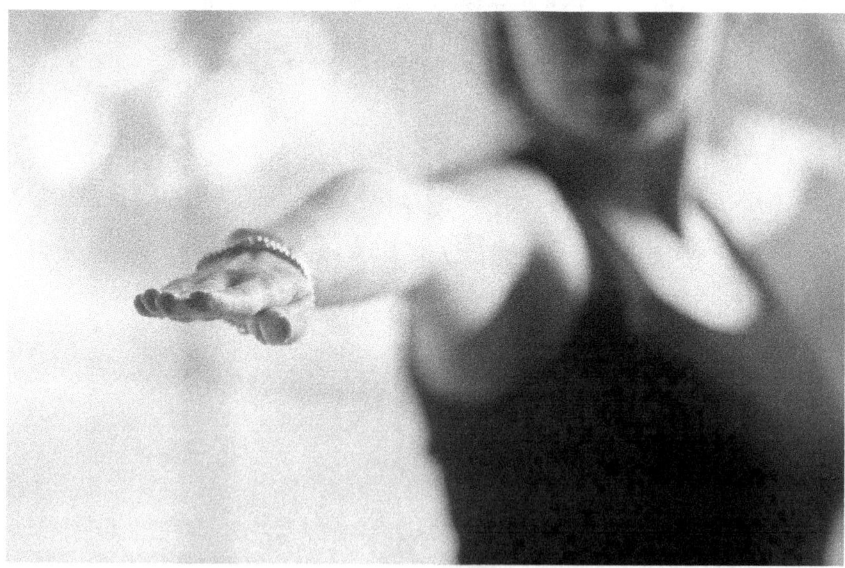

Arm Circles

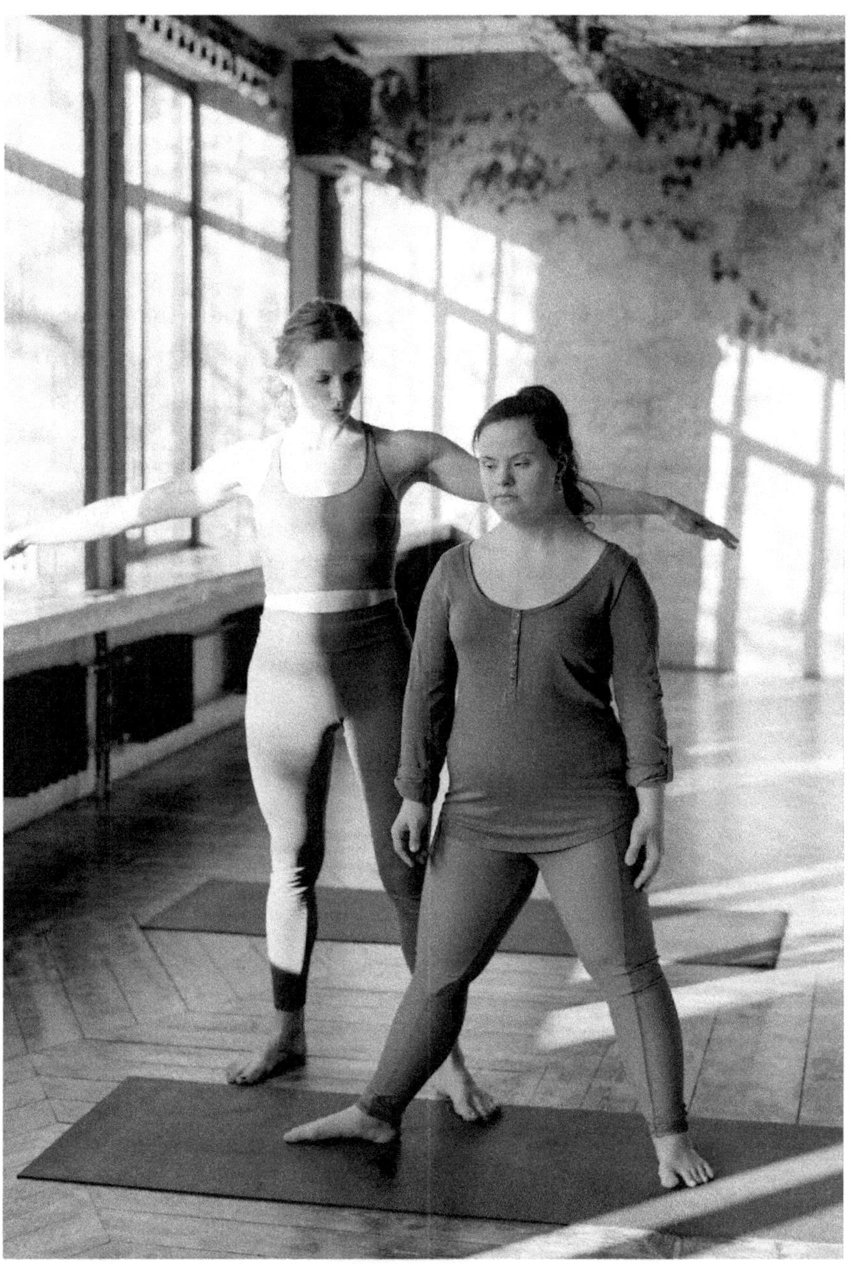

Arm Circles

WINDMILL TOE TOUCH

The windmill can be an aerobic exercise that also work your core and helps to tone the muscles in your lower body, chest, and shoulders.

- Begin standing with your feet spread slightly wider than your hips. Your arms will reach above your head and separate to form a Y.
- Bend at the waist while keeping your arms straight rotating to reach across your body with one hand to touch the opposite foot.
- This is an alternating toe touch, so after touching one foot, you will return to your starting position and repeat the movement to the opposite side. Repeat the steps for your desired amount of time or number of sets.

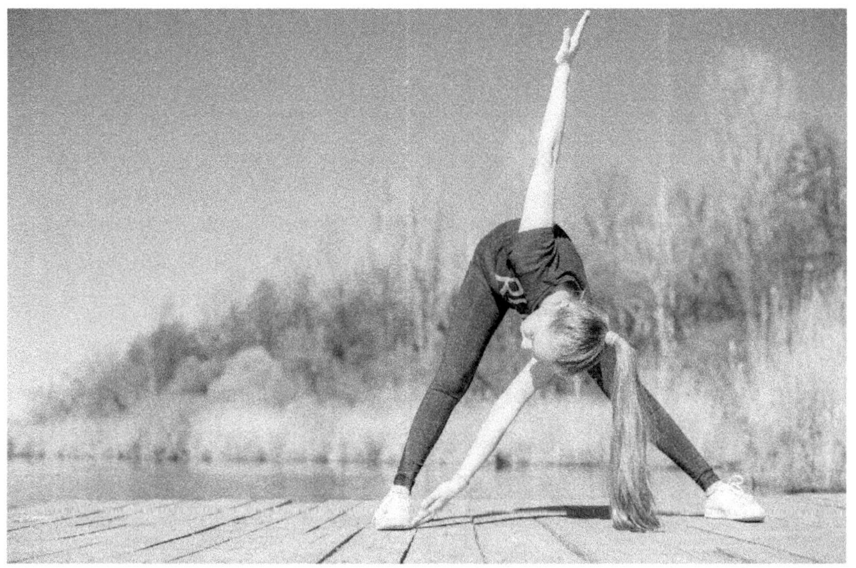

Windmill Toe Touch

CONCLUSION

There you have it, some of my very favorite exercises to do from the comfort of my living room. I like to choose five or six moves and do three sets of ten for each of them. Sometimes I do timed exercises where I choose a move to perform for 60 seconds before switching to another. If I am doing timed exercises, I try to again choose five or six and rotate every minute for anywhere between 10 and twenty minutes depending on my schedule and desired workout.

This is by no means an exhaustive list of all of the amazing options for exercise and fitness. This book is intended to be an introduction and hopefully a guide to some simple strategies for you to incorporate more movement in your day. I wanted this to include exercises that can be done in limited space with little to no equipment. I also wanted to include moves that would work multiple muscle groups in order to maximize the benefits you could gain in a short amount of time.

I hope that you are able to find benefit, enjoyment, and a new sense of motivation. If you do, I would greatly appreciate it if you could leave a positive review on Amazon.

PHOTO CREDITS/RESOURCES

PHOTO CREDITS

Stretches Title Page Photo by: Angela Roma (PEXELS)

Seated Neck Stretch **Photo by:** KoolShooters (PEXELS)

Lunging Calf Stretch Photo by: Andres Ayrton (PEXELS)

Cross Arm Stretch Photo by: Miriam Alonso (PEXELS)

Tricep Stretch Photo by: Ketut Subiyanto (PEXELS)

Supine Leg Stretch Photo By: https://www.freepik.com/free-photo/
woman-
practicing-advanced-
yoga-by-water_9344105.htm#page=2&query=leg%20
stretching&position=
3&from_view=keyword&track=ais&uuid=1dad68b8-0fa3-479d-
b0a2-a7d45f38e937

Standing Quad Stretch Photo by: Angela Roma (PEXELS)

Happy Baby Stretch Photo by: Vlada Karpovich (PEXELS)

Balance Title Page Photo by: Shvets Production (PEXELS)

Standing Balance Photo by: Cottonbro studio (PEXELS)

Prone 100 Photo By:
https://www.freepik.com/free-photo/sporty-woman-practicing
-yoga-back-buttock-training-pose-stretching-watching-fitness-
Video-tutorial-online-laptop-doing-workout-home-sitting-mat-
living-room-practicing_14779494.htm#query=glute%20bridge%

20with%20leg%20extension&position=49&from_view=search&track
=ais&uuid=122db1ab-1cae-4271-a7b2-a4682a7831da
Corkscrew Pilates Photo By:
https://www.freepik.com/free-photo/fit-young-woman-doing-
stretching-exercise-yoga-mat_3480237.htm#query=corkscrew
%20exercise&position=26&from_view=search&track=ais&uuid=
e66bf586-3235-432e-acdf-c6ec0a4cf9a3
Tree Pose Photo by: Cliff Booth (PEXELS)
Bird Dog Photo by: Cliff Booth (PEXELS)
Rotational Push Up Photo by: Marta Wave (PEXELS)
Strength Title Page Photo by: Anna Shvets (PEXELS)
Squats Photo by: Antoni Shkraba (PEXELS)
Frog Squat **Photo by: Ivan Samkov (PEXELS**
Planks Photo by: Mike GonzÃ¡lez (PEXELS)
Glute/Hamstring Bridge Photo By:
https://www.freepik.com/free-photo/young-woman-doing-yoga
-exercise-mat_3480247.htm#query=glute%20bridge%20up
&position=22&from_view=search&track=ais&uuid=a0e26b6d
-da56-445b-a806-e12b099a5d81
https://www.freepik.com/free-photo/full-shot-woman-doing
-yoga-seaside_22303246.htm#query=full-shot-woman-doing
-yoga-seaside&position=16&from_view=search&track=sph&uuid
=dd1039cd-78d1-40ff-89b2-89e9e432f48e
Fire Hydrant Photo by: Getty Images/iStockphoto
Donkey KIck Photo By:
https://www.freepik.com/free-photo/portrait-fitness-confident
-woman-black-sports-clothing-sexy-young-beautiful-model
-with-perfect-body-female-isolated-white-wall-studio-stretching
-out-before-training-raising-her-leg_25434867.htm#page=2&query
=Glute%20bridge%20with%20leg%20extension&position=12&from
_view=search&track=ais&uuid=fee2681b-68e9-4878-b4c6-

cea97b6ab4a8

Bicep Curl Photo by: Andrea Piacquadio (PEXELS)

Front Raises Photo by: Karolina Grabow (PEXELS)

Lateral Side Raises Photo by: Kampus Productions (PEXELS)

Tricep Extension Photo 1 By: Mike GonzÃ¡lez (PEXELS)

Photo 2 By: https://www.freepik.com/free-photo/attractive-athlet

e-

woman-isolated_9077452.htm#page=2&query=women%20
dumbbell%20overhead%20extension&position=39&from_
view=search&track=ais&uuid=91b61b85-dbaf-4d00-933d-
72a12d33a981

Aerobic Title Page Photo by: RDNE Stock (PEXELS)

Jump Rope Photo by: Mart Production (PEXELS)

March in Place Photo by: Polina Tankilevitch (PEXELS)

High Knees Photo by: Pavel Danilyuk (PEXELS)

Knees to Elbows Photo by: Dinielle De Veyra (PEXELS)

Arm Circle Photo 1 By:

https://www.freepik.com/free-photo/young-sporty-woman-
warrior-two-pose-studio-background_3939753.htm#query=arm
%20circling%20exercise&position=23&from_view=search&track
=ais&uuid=241f5e12-7b73-4b32-a02a-849eff494223

Photo 2 By: Photo by: Cliff Booth (PEXELS)

Windmill Toe Touch Photo By: https://www.freepik.com/free-phot

o/teenager-

warming-up

-pier_1574901.htm#query=alternating%20windmillexercise&position
=15&from_view=search&track=ais&uuid=9f25615a-ab54-4a97
-8c09-67af2f8f8462

RESOURCES

Goldman, R. (2020) *Leg stretches: Improve flexibility, Healthline.* Available at: https://www.healthline.com/health/exercise-fitness/leg-stretches-flexibility (Accessed: 16 February 2024).

AJ;, K.A. (2012) *Effect of acute static stretch on maximal muscle performance: A systematic review, Medicine and science in sports and exercise.* Available at: https://pubmed.ncbi.nlm.nih.gov/21659901/ (Accessed: 16 February 2024).

KOKKONEN, JOKE1; NELSON, ARNOLD G.2; ELDREDGE, CAROL1; WINCHESTER, JASON B.2. Chronic Static Stretching Improves Exercise Performance. Medicine & Science in Sports & Exercise 39(10):p 1825-1831, October 2007. | DOI: 10.1249/mss.0b013e3181238a2b

Best exercises for women over 50 (2019) *Gateway Region YMCA.* Available at: https://gwrymca.org/blog/best-exercises-women-over-50 (Accessed: 16 February 2024).

Taylor, P. (2019) *The 21 best stretching exercises for better flexibility, Stay Fit Master.* Available at: https://stayfitmaster.com/the-21-best-stretching-exercises-for-better-flexibility/ (Accessed: 16 February 2024).

Alexa Tucker, C.S. (2023) *11 calf stretches that will feel amazing if you've been sitting all day, SELF.* Available at: https://www.self.com/gallery/essential-calf-stretches (Accessed: 16 February 2024).

Wilkenson, A. (2021) 'Go With The Flow', *Woman's Health,* October.

Stobo, R. (2021) *How to reach the top of Tree pose (Vrksasana): The 411, Greatist.* Available at: https://greatist.com/fitness/tree-pose (Accessed:

16 February 2024).

Cronkleton, E. (2023) *Bird dog exercise: How to do, variations, and muscles targeted, Healthline*. Available at: https://www.healthline.com/health/bird-dog-exercise (Accessed: 16 February 2024).

Elina (2018) *Tutorial: How to perform the push-up with rotation, EVO Fitness*. Available at: https://evofitness.at/en/tutorial-push-up-with-rotation/ (Accessed: 16 February 2024).

Contributors, W.M. (2023) *Health Benefits of Squats, WebMD*. Available at: https://www.webmd.com/fitness-exercise/health-benefits-of-squats (Accessed: 16 February 2024).

JB;, K.J.A.C. (no date) *Chronic static stretching improves exercise performance, Medicine and science in sports and exercise*. Available at: https://pubmed.ncbi.nlm.nih.gov/17909411/ (Accessed: 16 February 2024).

Malia Frey, M.A. (2022) *How to do a triceps extension: Techniques, benefits, variations, Verywell Fit*. Available at: https://www.verywellfit.com/how-to-do-a-triceps-extension-techniques-benefits-variations-5082227 (Accessed: 16 February 2024).

Sayer, A. (2022) *Glute Bridge vs hip thrust: Which exercise is more effective?, Huy Hòa*. Available at: https://huyhoa.net/en/glute-bridge-vs-hip-thrust/ (Accessed: 16 February 2024).

Nunez, K. (2019) *Fire hydrant exercise: Technique, benefits, and tips, Healthline*. Available at: https://www.healthline.com/health/exercise-fitness/fire-hydrant-exercise (Accessed: 16 February 2024).

All, R. (2023, December 21). *20 cardio exercises to do at home with minimal equipment, from beginner to advanced.* https://www.medicalnewstoday.com/articles/cardio-exercises-at-home

Alleva, M. (2017, March 27). *Today's Workout: Windmill move good for stretching or as a warmup.* https://www.dispatch.com/story/lifestyle/health-fitness/2017/03/27/today-x2019-s-workout-windmill/21866747007/#.